INTRODUCTION TO PHARMACEUTICS – I

(According to P.C.I. Education Regulation — 1991)

INTRODUCTION TO PHARMACEUTICS – I

(According to P.C.I. Education Regulation – 1991)

ASHOK K. GUPTA
M. Pharm. (Pharmaceutics)
Head of Department, Pharmacy
Govt. Polytechnic for Women, Chandigarh

CBS

CBS Publishers & Distributors Pvt Ltd

New Delhi • Bengaluru Chennai Kochi Kolkata Lucknow Mumbai
Hyderabad Jharkhand Nagpur Patna Pune Uttarakhand

Introduction to
Pharmaceutics I
(According to PCI Education Regulation, 1991)
Third Edition

ISBN-13: 978-81-239-0273-9

Third Edition: 1994
Reprint: 1998, 1999, 2000, 2001, 2002, 2003, 2004, 2005, 2006, 2007, 2008, 2009, 2011, 2013, 2014, 2016, 2017, 2018, 2019, 2023, **2024**
First Edition: 1986
Second Edition: 1987
Reprint: 1989, 1992

Published by **Satish Kumar Jain** and produced by **Varun Jain** for

CBS Publishers & Distributors Pvt Ltd
4819/XI Prahlad Street, 24 Ansari Road, Daryaganj, New Delhi 110 002, India.
Ph: 011-23289259, 23266861 Website: www.cbspd.com
e-mail: delhi@cbspd.com

Corporate Office: 204 FIE, Industrial Area, Patparganj, Delhi 110 092
Ph: 011-4934 4934 Fax: 011-4934 4935
e-mail: publishing@cbspd.com; publicity@cbspd.com

Branches

- **Bengaluru:** Seema House 2975, 17th Cross, KR Road, Banasankari 2nd Stage, Bengaluru 560 070, Karnataka, India
  Ph: +91-80-26771678/79 Fax: +91-80-26771680 e-mail: bangalore@cbspd.com
- **Chennai:** 7, Subbaraya Street, Shenoy Nagar, Chennai 600 030, Tamil Nadu, India
  Ph: +91-44-26680620, 26681266 Fax: +91-44-42032115 e-mail: chennai@cbspd.com
- **Kochi:** 42/1325, 1326, Power House Road, Opp KSEB, Power House, Ernakulum Kochi 682 018, Kerala, India
  Ph: +91-484-4059061-65,67 Fax: +91-484-4059065 e-mail: kochi@cbspd.com
- **Kolkata:** 147, Hind Ceramics Compound, 1st Floor, Nilgunj Road, Belghoria, Kolkata-700056, West Bengal, India
  Ph: +033-25633055, 033-25633056 e-mail: kolkata@cbspd.com
- **Lucknow:** Basement, Khushnuma Complex, 7 Meerabai Marg (Behind Jawahar Bhawan), Lucknow-226001, UP, India
  Ph: +0522-4000032 e-mail: tiwari.lucknow@cbspd.com
- **Mumbai:** PWD Shed, Gala no 25/26, Ramchandra Bhatt Marg, Next to JJ Hospital Gate no. 2, Opp. Union Bank of India, Noorbaug, Mumbai-400009, Maharashtra, India
  Ph: 022-66661880/89 e-mail: mumbai@cbspd.com

Representatives

- Hyderabad 0-9885175004
- Jharkhand 0-9811541605
- Nagpur 0-8692091830
- Patna 0-9334159340
- Pune 0-9664372571
- Uttarakhand 0-9716462459

Printed at Glorious Printers, Jhilmil Industrial Area, Delhi, India

Preface to the Second Edition

The first edition of this book titled "Introduction to Pharmaceutics Part II", based on Education Regulation 1981 of Pharmacy Council of India was presented in the hands of the esteemed teachers and students of Diploma in Pharmacy in the year 1991. This book was warmly accepted and appreciated by the teachers as well as students of pharmacy throughout the country which gave a lot of satisfaction and encouragement. It inspired me to write the second edition according to Education Regulation 1991 titled "Introduction to Pharmaceutics I." I am highly thankful to all of them for the appreciation, healthy criticism and valuable suggestions.

Since the Pharmacy Council of India according to Education Regulation 1991 has recast the syllabus for Diploma in Pharmacy in which a large number of new topics like introduction to different dosage forms, drug delivery systems, Ayurvedic dosage forms, introduction to pharmacopoeias, micro-encapsulation etc has been incorporated, so it was necessary to bring this book upto the latest requirements of the teachers and students. Every effort has been made to present the material in a very precise manner covering all the topics prescribed by Pharmacy Council of India Education Regulation 1991.

The book is written in a very simple language giving suitable illustrations wherever required to make the students understand the topics in a better manner.

My sincere thanks are due to the learned teachers and students who has given me encouragement by warmly accepting the first edition and inspiring me for bringing out the second edition of this book. I hope this edition will also be warmly received and fulfil all the requirements of the teachers as well as students.

I owe a debt of gratitude to our ex-principal Sh. Jaishi Ram Bhardwaj and Sh. S.S. Bajaj, Head of Department of Pharmacy Govt. Polytechnic for Women Chandigarh for their elderly advice, encouragement, constructive criticism and guidance from time to time.

I am grateful to Sh. Satish Kumar Jain and M/s CBS publishers and distributors for bringing out this edition in a short span of time.

I will be thankful to the teachers and students for their valuable criticism and suggestions for improving the quality of the book

A.K. GUPTA

Preface to the First Edition

The author feel great pleasure in presenting this book titled 'Introduction to Pharmaceutics part II' in the hands of the esteemed teachers and students of Diploma in Pharmacy.

With the introduction of Education Regulation 1981 of Pharmacy Council of India, the course contents of Diploma in Pharmacy were revised to meet the present day requirements of the industries and practising pharmacists. Since no book is available which fulfil all the requirements therefore the author has ventured to write this book covering all the topics of the new syllabus to meet the long felt demand of the teachers and students of Diploma in Pharmacy. Taking into consideration the difficulties faced by the students this book is written strictly according to the syllabus and in a simple language giving suitable illustrations where applicable. I am confident that they would like the book.

I am deeply indebted to our Ex-principal Sh. J.R. Bhardwaj for inspiration, guidance and elderly advice from time to time.

My sincere thanks are due to Sh. S.S. Bajaj, Head of Department of Pharmacy Govt. Polytechnic for Women Chandigarh for the encouragement, constructive criticism and guidance he has been giving whenever any problem was discussed with him.

I owe a debt of gratitude to my colleagues and friends teaching in different pharmacy institutions throughout the country for promptly responding to the request for providing information on different aspects of the subject matter of the book.

I am thankful to Sh. Satish Kumar Jain and M/s CBS publishers and distributors for taking out present book in a commendably short time inspite of heavy seasonal work.

Inspite of geat care there may be mistakes and deficiencies. I will be grateful to the teachers and students who point them out and make suggestions for improving the quality of the book.

AUGUST 1991 A.K. GUPTA

Contents

1
Pharmaceutical Dosage Forms and New Drug Delivery Systems

The following are short descriptions of pharmaceutical dosage forms and preparations that may be dispensed in the hospital pharmacy or on the retail counter.

Aerosols

The term aerosol has a specific meaning denoting a fine dispersion of liquid or solid particles in a gas where the particle size is less than 50 µm in diameter, as in the case of mist or smoke.

Aerosols may be defined as the pressurised dosage form of medicament in which the liquid or solid drug or drugs are dissolved or suspended in gas. The gas used for this purpose is known as propellant. The aerosols are packed in a suitable container known as aerosol container, when pressure is applied to the aerosol system, the contents are expelled out through the opening of the valve in the form of mist, a coarse, wet or dry spray, a stream or as a foam. The aerosols used in the treatment of respiratory conditions, are atomised in devices known as atomisers or nebulisers. The type of atomiser used depends upon the viscosity of the spray solution, the more viscous the solution, the more powerful the atomiser needed.

Now a days pharmaceutical aerosols are frequently used both orally and topically to dispense a large number of drugs including local analgesics, antiseptics, fungicidal agents, antibiotics and anti-inflamatory agents etc. A number of veterinary and pet products have also been put into aerosol dosage forms. A variety of non-pharmaceutical preparations such as personal deodorant sprays, cosmetic hair sprays, perfume sprays, shaving lathers, tooth paste and various house hold products such as spray starch, waxes, polishes, cleansers and lubricants are available as aerosols.

The potent drugs used for the relief of asthma are dissolved or suspended in a suitable solvent or propellant and are enclosed in a container which is fitted with a metering device that delivers a measured dose. Drugs administered in this way give rapid response and quick onset of action as compared with drugs administered orally. But the frequent use of such inhalations or sprays are not without risk and adverse reactions. Therefore it is advisable to warn the patient to strictly follow the directions given by the doctor and frequent use of such preparations should be avoided.

Aerosol containers provide a number of advantages over the more traditional methods of presentation of drugs that they are compact, convenient to carry and easy to apply evenly without touching the painful surfaces. A measured amount of drug and uniform doses are administered by metered valves. The product remains free from contamination and sterility of the preparation is maintained as no micro-organisms can enter the pack when the valve is opened. They also provide good protection from oxidation and light to those drugs which are destroyed by air and light. Hydrolysis of drugs is prevented since the propellants contain no water. Because the filling and sealing of pressurised aerosols require special machinery and techniques therefore these preparations are costlier than traditional dosage forms.

Applications

Applications are liquid or viscous preparations intended for application to the skin. Usually, they are suspensions or emulsions. Most of the official preparations contain parasiticides and are intended for only a limited number of applications.

They should be dispensed in coloured fluted bottles in order to distinguish them from preparations meant for internal use. The container should be labelled "for external use only" Examples of applications are calamine application compound, B.P.C., dicophane application, B.P.C.

Aromatic Waters

Aromatic waters are also known as medicated waters. They are dilute, usually saturated, aqueous solutions of volatile oils or volatile substances. Some of them have a mild therapeutic action but mainly they are used as flavouring agents in preparations meant for internal administration of drugs. Aromatic waters may be prepared either by diluting the concentrated waters or by shaking the volatile substances with water. Aromatic waters include anise water, camphor water, chloroform water, cinnamon water and peppermint water.

Cachets

Cachets consists of a dry powder enclosed in a shell, usually prepared from a mixture of rice flour and water by moulding into a suitable shape and drying. They are quite useful for administering the drugs with unpleasant taste and a large dose can be enclosed in a cachet than in a tablet or capsule.

There are two kinds of cachets; 'wet seal' cachets which are sealed by moistening the edges with water, and 'dry seal' cachets.

Before administration, a cachet should be immersed in water for a few seconds, then placed on the tongue and swallowed with a draught of water. Cachets should be stored and supplied in well closed air tight containers. Examples are sodium aminosalicylate cachets, sodium aminosalicylate and isoniazid cachets.

Capsules

Capsules are the solid unit dosage form of medicament in which the drug or drugs are enclosed in a practically tasteless, hard or soft soluble container or shell made up of a suitable form of gelatin. Hard capsules are used for filling the solid substances. Hard gelatin capsules are available in a number of sizes which varies from 000 to 5, the former being the largest and latter the smallest. They are made up of two cylindrical halves, one slightly larger in diameter but shorter in length known as cap and the other slightly shorter in diameter but longer in length know as base. the medicament is filled in longer narrower half, then the cap is fitted over the open end by moistening edges of the lower half of the capsule.

Soft capsules are flexible in nature. They may be spherical, ovoid, cylindrical or tubes. The spherical capsules are also known as 'Pearls'. Soft gelatin capsules are used for enclosing the solids, liquids and semi-liquids.

Enteric coated capsules are the capsules which are treated or coated in such a way that the capsule does not disintegrate in the acidic medium of the stomach but disintegrate in the alkaline medium of the small intestine. Enteric coated capsules have been largely replaced by enteric coated tablets.

Capsules are increasing their popularity day by day. Hard capsule comes second to tablets in importance as solid unit dosage forms. Some of the capsules are administered through rectum and vagina and are convenient mode of administration of drugs than suppositories. For oral administration the capsule is placed on the tongue and swallowed with a drink of water.

Collodions

Collodions are the liquid preparations meant for external application to the skin. They are convenient applications for small cuts and abrasions and are also used when a prolonged contact between the skin and the medicament is required. The vehicle used is volatile and evaporates on application to skin, leaving a flexible, protective film covering at the site of application. They are applied with a brush or rod.

Flexible collodion contains pyroxillon, castor oil and alcohol in solvent ether. Alcohol and solvent ether are used as vehicle, pyroxillon as film producing agent and castor oil gives flexibility.

Creams

Creams are viscous semisolid emulsions intended for application to the skin. Creams differ from ointments that they have lighter body than ointments. Moreover due to the presence of water soluble bases they can be easily removed from skin and clothings. Creams may be of oil in water (aqueous creams) or water in oil (oily creams) type. The aqueous creams have a tendency to bacterial and mold growth, therefore a preservative must be added in their formulation. Examples are cetomacrogol cream, cetrimide cream, chlorhexidine cream, hydrocortisone cream etc.

Draughts (Haustus)

A draught is a liquid oral preparation taken as a single dose. If several doses are prescribed, each dose is dispensed in separate container. Ipecacuanha Emetic Draught, Paediatric; is an exception where several doses are prescribed in a multiple-dose container. Examples are : male fern extract draught and paraldehyde draught.

Dusting Powders

Dusting powders are meant for external application to the skin. They are usually mixtures of two or more than two ingredients in fine powder e.g. starch, kaolin, talc, zinc oxide etc. They must be homogeneous and in a very fine state of subdivision to enhance effectiveness and minimise local irritation, for this purpose they may be passed through sieve no 120. Dusting powders are applied to the skin for antiseptic, antipruritic, astringent, antiperspirant, absorbent, protective and lubricant purposes.

Dusting powders are dispensed in sifter-top containers or pressure aerosols. They may also be supplied in wide mouth containers and applied with powder puff, a soft brush or a sterile gauge pad but care must be taken to avoid mechanical irritation to the skin surface. Dusting powders should not be applied to open wounds or to raw surfaces. Examples are : dicophane dusting powder, zinc and salicylic acid dusting powder; zinc, starch and talc dusting powder.

Dentifrices

Dentifrices are substances or preparations which are generally used with the help of tooth brush for cleaning the surfaces of the teeth. They are available in the form of fine powders and pastes.

Ear Drops

Ear drops are the liquid preparations in which the drug or drugs are dissolved or suspended in a suitable vehicle like water, dilute alcohol, glycerin or propylene glycol and are intended for instillation into the ear with a dropper. They are generally used for cleansing the ear, drying weeping surfaces, softening the wax and for treating the mild infections.

Ear drops are dispensed in coloured, fluted bottles attached with a dropper or in suitable plastic containers. The containers should be labelled "for external use only". Examples are : hydrogen peroxide ear drops, phenol ear drops etc.

Elixirs

Elixirs are clear, pleasantly flavoured, sweetened hydroalcoholic liquid preparations for oral administration. The main ingredients of elixirs are ethanol and water but glycerin, sorbitol, propylene glycol, flavouring agents, sugar and preservatives may be incorporated to the preparation. The elixirs may be medicated or non-medicated. The medicated elixirs usually contain very potent drugs such as antibiotics, antihistaminics and sedatives. The non-medicated elixirs are used as flavours and vehicles. Examples are : chlorpheniramine elixir, diphenhydramine elixir, ephedrine elixir, paracetamol elixir, paediatric; piperazine citrate elixir etc.

Emulsions

Emulsions are the biphasic liquid dosage form of medicament in which two immiscible liquids (generally one of which is water and the other is some lipid or oil) are made miscible by the addition of a third substance known as emulgent or emulsifying agent. Emulsions are comparatively pleasant to take than to take an oil as such.

Emulsions are of two types (a) oil in water type (O/W) (b) water in oil type (W/O). The former is generally for oral administration whereas the latter is generallv for application to the skin.

Emulsions should be supplied in wide mouthed containers labelled with "shake the bottle before use" label. Examples of emulsion are : castor oil emulsion, liquid paraffin emulsion, liquid paraffin and phenolphthalein emulsion etc.

Enemas

Enemas are aqueous or oily solutions or suspensions intended for introduction into the rectum for their purgative, sedative, anthelmintic, anti-inflammatory or nutritive effects. They may also be used for X-ray examination of the lower bowel. Among the commonly used drugs in solution form which act as cleansing enemas include isotonic solution of sodium chloride, sodium bicarbonate 2%, sodium phosphate, magnesium sulphate, soap and a combination of these substances. The other drugs in the form of enemas include olive oil, arachis oil, chloralhydrate, paraldehyde, turpentine, alum, tannic acid, barium sulphate etc.

Usually solutions in volume of 500 ml to 1000 ml, depending on the age and condition of the patient is introduced as enema. However the commercially available concentrated enemas are introduced in small volumes of 100 to 200 ml. Large volume enemas should be warmed to body temperature before administration. Examples are : paraldehyde enema, soap enema etc.

Eye Drops

Eye drops are sterile aqueous or oily solutions or suspensions for instillation into the eye. They are usually applied into the space between the eye ball and eyelids or on to the corneal surface. The main requirement of eye drops is that they should be sterile, usually isotonic, buffered and free from foreign particles to avoid irritation to the eye. They usually contain substances having antiseptic, anaesthetic, anti-inflammatory, mydriatic or miotic properties or substances used for diagnostic purposes.

Eye drops should be dispensed in glass or suitable plastic containers with a screw cap fitted with a rubber teat and glass dropper for easy application of the drops or the containers may be fitted with a narrow nozzle from which the drops can be directly instilled into the eye. Examples are : atropine eye drops, chloramphenicol eye drops, cocaine eye drops, hydrocortisone eye drops, hyoscine eye drops, pilocarpine eye drops, sulphacetamide eye drops etc.

Eye lotions

Eye lotions or eye washes are sterile aqueous solutions used for irrigating the eye. They are usually applied with a clean eye bath or sterile fabric dressing and a large volume of solution is allowed to flow quickly over the eye.

Eye lotions are usually supplied in concentrated form and are required to be diluted with an equal volume of warm water immediately before use. They should be freshly prepared and should not be stored for more than 2-3 days as they may be contaminated with micro-organisms on prolonged storage. Eye lotions should be isotonic and free from foreign particles to avoid irritation to the eye. The drugs used for preparing eye solutions include sodium chloride, sodium bicarbonate, boric acid, borax and zinc sulphate.

Eye lotions should be dispensed in coloured fluted bottles. The container should be labelled "for external use only". Examples are : sodium bicarbonate eye lotion and sodium chloride eye lotion.

Gargles

Gargles are aqueous solutions used for the prevention or treatment of throat infections. Usually they are concentrated solutions and should be diluted with warm water before use. In using the gargles they are brought into intimate contact with the mucous membrane of the throat and are allowed to remain there for a few moments after which they are thrown out of the mouth. Some of the analgesic preparations like aspirin gargles may be swallowed afterwards.

Gargles should be dispensed in white fluted bottles.

Gels

Generally gels are the aqueous colloidal suspensions of the hydrated forms of insoluble inorganic drugs. Examples are aluminium hydroxide gel, aluminium phosphate gel, milk of magnesia etc. They are generally used as antacid.

Glycerins

They are also known as glycerites. Glycerins are the viscous preparations in which the drug is dissolved in glycerin with or without heating. They are generally used as antiseptic or anti-inflammatory preparations. Examples are ichthammol glycerin, phenol glycerin, tannic acid glycerin etc.

Granules

Granules are the solid dosage form of medicament in which the powdered drug or drugs are mixed with sweetening, flavouring and colouring agents. A suitable granulating agent is added to moisten the powder and mixed thoroughly. The wet mass is passed through a suitable sieve and granules dried at a temperature of 60°C. They are supplied in glass containers and the patient is asked to add sufficient freshly boiled and cooled water to constitute a liquid preparation.

Effervescent Granules

These are specially prepared solid dosage form of medicament, meant for internal use. They usually contain citric acid, tartaric acid, sodium bicarbonate and medicament, a sweetening agent such as saccharin or sucrose may be incorporated.

When these granules are added to water, the acids react with sodium bicarbonate to librate carbon dioxide and the preparation is taken while effervescing or immediately afterwards. These preparations act as antacid.

Implants

Implants are sterile small tablets meant for insertion under the skin by giving a small cut into the skin which is stitched afterwards. They are used to provide slow and continuous release of the drug for a long time ranging from 3 to 6 months or even more. These tablets are more commonly used in animals than human beings. Generally steroidal hormones like testosterone, stilbesterol etc. are formulated as implants.

Infusions

Infusions are liquid preparations which are either prepared by infusion process or by diluting 1 part of concentrated infusion with 9 parts of water. Infusions should be freshly prepared and must be used within 12 hours of their preparation. Examples are concentrated compound gentian infusion and concentrated senega infusion.

Inhalations

Inhalations are the liquid preparations containing volatile ingredients. They are used to relieve nasal congestion and inflammation of the respiratory tract. They may be placed on a pad or added to hot water and vapours inhaled for five to ten minutes. Examples are benzoin inhalation, menthol and eucalyptus inhalation.

Injections

Injections are the sterile liquid preparations containing one or more medicaments dissolved or suspended in a suitable vehicle and are meant for introduction into the body tissues by means of an injection under or through one or more layers of the skin or mucous membrane. Examples are ampicillin injection, dextrose intravenous infusion, gentamycin injection etc.

Insufflations

These are the finely divided powders meant for introduction into the body cavities such as ears, nose, tooth sockets and vagina with the help of an apparatus known as insufflator, to which it would be difficult to apply the powder directly.

Irrigations

These are the solutions containing medicaments used to treat infections of the bladder, vagina and nose. These are introduced into the cavities by means a soft rubber tube known as catheter. They are generally used as antiseptic, anti-inflammatory or cleansing solutions.

Jellies

Jellies are transparent or translucent non-greasy semisolid preparations meant for external application to the skin or mucous membrane. They are used for medication or lubrication purposes. Some of them are also used as contraceptive jellies. Examples are proflavin jelly, ichthammol jelly etc.

Linctuses

Linctuses are sweet, viscous liquid preparations usually containing medicinal substances which have demulcent, sedative or expectorant properties. They are used for the treatment of cough. Linctuses are swallowed slowly in small doses without addition of water. Examples are codeine linctus, noscapine linctus etc.

Liniments

Liniments are liquid or semiliquid preparations meant for external application to the skin. Liniments are applied by rubbing or friction but should not be applied to the broken skin. They should be dispensed in coloured fluted bottles in order to distinguish from preparations meant for external use. The bottle should be labelled "for external use only" and "shake the bottle before use". Examples are soap liniment, white liniment etc.

Lotions

Lotions are liquid suspensions or dispersions meant for external application to the skin without friction. They usually contain alcohol and glycerin because alcohol hastens drying and produces cooling sensation whereas glycerin keeps the skin moist for a sufficient long time.

Lotions should be dispensed in a coloured fluted bottle with "for external use only" and "shake the bottle before use" label. Examples are calamine lotion and salicylic acid lotion.

Lozenges

Lozenges are the solid dosage form of medicament which are meant for slow dissolution in the mouth. Along with medicament they contain a sweetening agent, flavouring agent and a strong binding agent. They may be prepared either by moulding or by compression. Examples are compound bismuth lozenges, liquorice lozenges etc.

Mixtures

Mixtures are liquid dosage form of medicament in which drug or drugs are dissolved or suspended in a suitable aqueous vehicle, they may be sweetened and flavoured. They are freshly prepared and consumed within a few days. Mixtures are meant for oral administration and generally several doses are contained in a bottle, when only one dose is there it is known as haustus or draught.

For indiffusible solids a suitable suspending agent will have to be incorporated to make the substance diffusible, so as to measure the dose easily. The containers of such mixtures should be labelled "shake the bottle before use". Examples are aluminium hydroxide mixture, kaolin mixture, magnesium sulphate mixture etc.

Mouthwashes

Mouthwashes are usually aqueous solutions in concentrated form with a pleasant taste and flavour used for rinsing, deodorant, refreshing or antiseptic action. Medicated mouthwashes may contain astringents, antibacterial agents, protein precipitants or other agents. They are generally used after dilution with warm water, on the mucous membrane of the mouth. Examples are compound sodium chloride mouthwash and zinc sulphate and zinc chloride mouthwash.

Nasal drops

Nasal drops are usually aqueous solutions intended for instillation into the nostrils by means of a dropper. They are commonly used for their antiseptic, local analgesic or vasoconstrictor properties. Examples are ephedrine nasal drops.

Ointments

Ointments are the soft semisolid preparations meant for external application to the skin or mucous membrane. They usually contain a medicament dissolved, suspended or emulsified in the base. Ointments are used for their emollient and protective action to the skin. Examples are compound benzoic acid ointment, calamine ointment, cetrimide emulsifying ointment etc.

Ophthalmic Ointments

Ophthalmic ointments are meant for application to the eye. They should be sterile and free from irritation. They should be packed in sterile containers which should keep the preparation sterile until whole of it is used up. Examples are atropine eye ointment, chloromycetin eye ointment.

Paints

Paints are the liquid preparations meant for external application to the skin or mucous membrane. They generally have a volatile solvent which evaporates quickly to leave a dry film of the medicament. Throat paints are viscous preparations which are applied to the throat. They contain high contents of glycerin due to which the preparations remain sticking to the site of application and prolong the action of the medicament. Examples are coal tar paint, compound iodine paint.

Pastes

Pastes are semisolid preparations meant for external application to the skin. They differ from ointments in that they generally contain a large amount of finely powdered solids such as starch, zinc oxide, calcium carbonate etc. They provide a protective coating over the areas to which they are applied. They may be applied directly to the affected part or by spreading on a suitable backing material which is then applied to the affected area. Examples are magnesium sulphate paste, zinc and coal tar paste.

Pessaries

Pessaries are the solid unit dosage form of medicament meant for introduction into the vagina. The bases used for the manufacture of pessaries are such that at room temperature they retain the original shape but when inserted into the cavity either melt or dissolve in the cavity fluids to release the medicament. They may be prepared either by moulding or by compression. Examples are lactic acid pessaries, nystatin pessaries.

Powders

Powders are solid dosage form of medicament meant for internal and external use. The powders meant for internal use are known as oral powders whereas those meant for external use are known as dusting powders. The powders may be simple or compound. When the powders are dispensed in large quantities in a container and the patient is asked to measure a specified quantity as a dose then these powders are known as bulk powders. Examples are compound rhubarb oral powder, compound sodium chloride and dextrose oral powder, talc dusting powder etc.

Solutions

Solutions are liquid preparations meant for internal or external use. They contain one or more than one ingredient usually dissolved in water. They may be sterile when intended for parenteral administration or unsterilized when intended for oral administration. Examples are strong ammonium acetate solution, aqueous iodine solution, cetrimide solution etc.

Solution tablets

Solution tablets contain a medicament or medicaments required to dissolve completely in the liquid to produce solutions of definite concentration. The solutions prepared by dissolving the soluble tablets may include mouthwashes, gargles, skin lotions, douches, antibiotics and certain vitamins. Examples are effervescing mouthwash tablets, benzyl penicillin solution tablets.

Spirits

Spirits are solutions of medicament or medicaments in alcohol (90 per cent). Examples are chloroform spirit, lemon spirit, compound orange spirit.

Sprays

Sprays are the liquid preparations of medicaments in aqueous, alcoholic or glycerin containing vehicle and are meant for application to the nose or throat by means of an atomiser or nebuliser. Examples are compound adrenaline and atropine spray, isoprenaline spray.

Suppositories

Suppositories are special shaped solid dosage form of medicament for insertion into body cavities other than mouth. They may be inserted into rectum, vagina or urethra. These products are so formulated that after insertion, they will either melt or dissolve in the cavity fluids to release the medicament. Suppositories vary in shapes, sizes and weights. Generally suppositories from 1 to 2 gm are prepared with either cocoa butter or glycerogelatin base. Examples are aminophylline suppositories, glycerol suppositories etc.

Suspensions

Suspensions are the biphasic liquid dosage form of medicament in which the finely divided solid particles ranging from 0.5 to 5.0 micron are suspended or dispersed in a liquid or semisolid vehicle. Suspensions are mainly used for oral administration, external application or parenteral use. Examples are barium sulphate suspension; chalk, kaolin suspension.

Syrups

Syrups are sweet, viscous, concentrated aqueous solutions of sucrose or other sugars in water or any other suitable aqueous vehicle. They are used as sweetening and flavouring agents. Examples are lemon syrup, raspberry syrup, tolu syrup etc.

Tablets

Tablets are unit solid dosage form of medicament or medicaments with or without suitable diluents. They are prepared by moulding or usually by compression. Tablets are generally meant for oral administration but may be used by other routes of administration. Examples are aminophylline tablets, chloroquine sulphate tablets, paracetamol tablets etc.

Tinctures

Tinctures are alcoholic liquid preparations containing the active principles of vegetable drugs. They are usually prepared by maceration or percolation, or may be prepared by dissolving the corresponding liquid extract or chemical substances in alcohol or hydroalcoholic solvent. Examples are belladonna tincture, aromatic cardamom tincture, nux vomica tincture etc.

Throat paints

Throat paints are viscous liquid preparations used for mouth and throat infections. Glycerin is commonly used as a base because of viscous nature and agreeable taste. Examples are boroglycerin, phenol glycerin and compound iodine paint (Mandl's paint).

DRUG DELIVERY SYSTEMS

With the advancement of technology, emerging concepts, new theories and their practical applications in the development and production of previously termed as "dosage forms" are now more appropriately referred to as "drug delivery systems."

With the development of new drug delivery systems, new drugs were discovered. The production processes, machines for manufacture, new control methods for accurate definition of drug delivery and new and improved quality control procedures were developed. All these changes and improvements lead to the production of superior quality drug dosage forms at lesser costs. With the development of new techniques, processes and instruments like microprocessors and small computers, the production of modern drugs has further been revolutionized to a great extent.

Majority of the drugs are administered to the body with the basic aim to achieve a stable blood or tissue concentration which is therapeutically effective and nontoxic for an extended period of time. This can only be achieved if proper dosage regimens are designed and attempt is made to attain a maximum rate and extent of drug absorption, however drug action can be controlled through formulation by controlling bioavailability to reduce drug absorption rates. By the use of new drug delivery systems one can enhance the bioavailability and therapeutic index of medicinal agents as well as reduce side effects and can improve acceptance and compliance by the patient. Following approaches to the formulation of drug delivery systems based on the deliberate control of drug availability are considered.

Sustained release, sustained action, prolonged action, extended action, controlled release, timed release, depot and repository dosage forms are terms used to identify drug delivery systems. These preparations are designed to achieve a prolonged therapeutic effect by continuously releasing the drug over an extended period of time after administration of a single dose of the drug. Now a days a large number of products are available in the market which are formulated for oral, parenteral, ophthalmic, transdermal, intravaginal and intrauterine administrations which act as sustained or controlled drug delivery systems. Research is being carried out to develop intranasal and rectal routes of administration.

Sustained release or controlled release drug delivery systemsw are found more suitable for the treatment of chronic diseases which require a prolonged use of drugs. Some of the diseases which require such type of treatment include : asthma, diabetes, hypertension, peptic ulcer, rheumatoid arthritis, cancer, angina pectoris, depression, anxiety, bacterial infections etc.

1. Oral Drug Delivery Systems

Sustained action dosage form of medicament like tablets and capsules are meant for oral administration and release the drug slowly and continuously for a prolonged duration of action, thus maintaining a minimum effective connectration (MEC) of the drug in the blood at a constant level throughout the treatment period. Whereas in the conventional therapy i.e. administration of the drug in divided doses at a specified intervals of time, a constant blood concentration is not maintained but there is a considerable fluctuation in drug concentration. Graphically these two types of concentrations can be represented as follows :

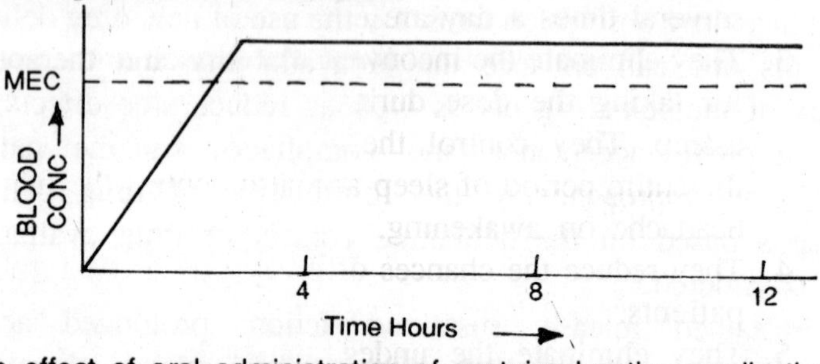

The effect of oral administration of sustained action medication.

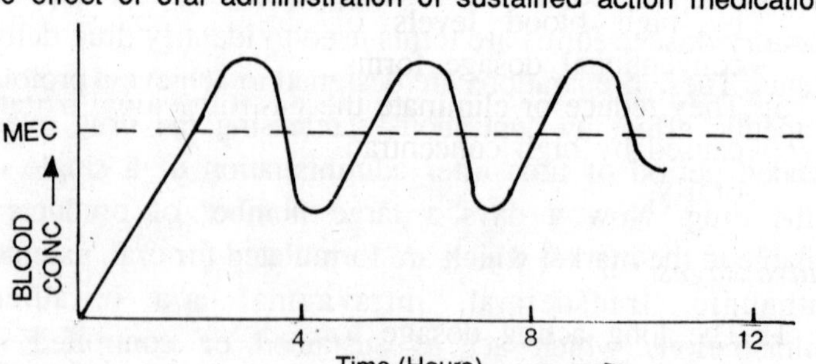

The effect of oral administration of medication in divided doses.

The sustained release or sustained action dosage forms release the initial dose immediately to cause a rapid onset of desired therapeutic action and the subsequent doses are released to maintain an effective concentration of the drug for the duration of the treatment. The initial desired therapeutic response is maintained because the rate of release of the desired therapeutic concentration is equal to the rate at which the drug is eliminated or inactivated. The products which release the drug for prolonged action are becoming more popular and are referred to as sustained-action, sustained-release, prolonged-action, prolonged-release, timed-release or repeat action products.

Advantages

1. They maintain the therapeutic effect for a longer period than obtained by the administration of single dose medication.
2. They are considered the most convenient dosage forms because the necessity of administering the doses serveral times a day are eliminated.
3. They eliminate the inconvenience caused to the patient for taking the dose during night hours when he is asleep. They control the level of sleep throughout the entire period of sleep and also control the migrain headache on awakening.
4. They reduce the chances of missed doses by forgetful patients.
5. They eliminate the undesirable side effects caused by high blood levels of drugs administered as conventional dosage forms.
6. They reduce or eliminate the gastrointestinal irritation caused by high concentrations of drugs administered orally.

Disadvantages

1. The long acting dosage forms may not release the drug as completely or effectively as those of conventional dosage forms.

2. Certain drugs are no more effective when administered in long acting forms.
3. They are comparatively costlier than the drugs in conventional dosage forms.

Principles Involved in the Development of Sustained Action Dosage Forms

When the drug is administered into the body, it is absorbed into the blood stream from the site of absorption, distributed, metabolised and eliminated out of the body in the original form or in the metabolised form. The amount of drug present in the circulation at any given time depends upon the rate of absorption, rate of biotransformation and rate of elimination of the drug. Thus the action of a drug can be prolonged by :

1. Decreasing the rate of absorption.
2. Decreasing the rate of biotransformation.
3. Decreasing the rate of excretion.

Out of the above mentioned factors, for the development of sustained action dosage forms it is not possible to either decrease the rate of biotransformation or the rate of elimination of drugs because both the factors involve the simultaneous administration of enzymes and other substances which interfere with the normal metabolic functions, therefore, cannot be administered. Thus the only factor which can be manipulated is to decrease the rate of absorption of drugs.

Design of Sustained Action Dosage Forms

It is the principle of sustained action dosage forms that the initial dose must be released immediately to the system to produce rapid action and the subsequent doses are released gradually and continuously at a specified time to maintain an effective blood concentration to produce the desired therapeutic effect for a specified period of time. Therefore the products so designed should conform to these requirements. Following are a few types of sustained action dosage forms generally used for the administration of drugs.

1. Coated Beads or Granules

The total quantity of the drug is divided into a suitable number of groups (generally 10 groups of pellets, 1-2 mm in diameter). The first group is kept uncoated to produce the rapid therapeutic effect and the other groups are coated with selected materials one by one to produce thickness of varying degrees. This can be done by giving two coating to the 2nd group, three coating to the 3rd group, four to the fourth and so on. The total thickness of these coatings should be about 0.1 mm. All these groups i.e. coated and uncoated are then mixed together. They may be compressed into tablets, filled in capsules or suspended in suitable liquids to produce liquid dosage forms. For coating, the materials may include cellulose esters, fats, keratin, and gluten. The other coating materials are mixtures of bees wax, carnuba wax with glyceryl monostearate. Stearic acid, palmitic acid and cetyl alcohol can also be used for coatings. Generally for coaring, beads of 12 to 40 mesh size are recommended and coating pans are used for coating the beads.

If the dose of the drug is small, then the blank granules or beads may be prepared from any inert material like lactose, starch or sucrose and the drug adsorbed on to them by dissolving the drug in a nonaqueous solvent mixture such as alcohol and acetone.

2. Matrix Embedding

In this process the drug is suspended in a melt of some water insoluble material such as carnauba wax or hydrogenated castor wax and the admixture is allowed to cool and solidify. The solidified mass is then ground to produce granules or coarse powder which can be used to prepare compressed tablets or filled into capsules. The grinding process often produces enough surface drug which is sufficient to release the initial dose. Too much grinding should be avoided because this may lead to uncover the drug thus rendering the embedding useless. The additional uncoated drug can be incorporated to release the initial dose immediately to produce the rapid therapeutic effect.

The inert, non-absorbable plastic materials such as polyvinyl chloride or ethylcellusose etc. can be used as matrix. The drug is mixed with the plastic materials and made in the form of granules or coarse powders which are then compressed or filled into capsules. Some channeling agents can be included which will help the drug to leach out of the matrix by body fluids and absorbed into the system, the plastic material remains unchanged and is excreted as such through the faeces.

3. Slowly Soluble Chemical Complex Formation

Some medicaments which possess very low solubilities may themselves act as sustained action preparation but the drugs which are very soluble may be chemically converted to complex forms which dissolve slowly thus acting as sustained action preparations. Griseofulvin, possess this property itself, whereas certain amine drugs combine with high molecular weight acids like tannic acid and polygalacturonic acid to form slightly soluble complexes which dissolve slowly in the body fluids thus increasing the time of release of the drug.

4. Use of Ion Exchange Resins

There are two types of ion exchange resins, one is known as cation or acid exchange resin and the other anion or base exchange resin. The cation exchange resin exchanges the cations in solution with hydrogen ions from resin whereas anion exchange resin removes the anions from resin. When a solution of the cationic drug is passed through the cation resin it forms a complex which is then washed with deionised water and compressed in the form oif tablets or filled into capsules. It may be dissolved in a suitable liquid to prepare a liquid dosage form. Before compression or filling into capsules a certian quantity of unbound drug sufficient to produce minimum effective concentration is incorporated to the resin complex. After administration the drug is released in greater amount in the acidic medium of the stomach than the alkaline medium of the small intestine.

Other Techniques of Producing Sustained Action of Drugs

The following are the other techniques by which sustained action of drugs can be produced.

1. Route of Administration

The absorption of a drug depends on the route by which it is administered. If it is administered by intravenous injection an immediate effect is produced whereas the effect is delayed if the sme drug in introduced by intramuscular injection. The effect can be prolonged which may last for months if the drug is placed under the skin as implant. Hence the route of administration can be used to produce sustained action of a drug.

2. Particle Size of the Drugs

Since the dissolution rate of a drug depends on its particle size the smaller the particle size more will be dissolution rate and bigger the particle size less will be dissolution rate. The absorption depends upon the dissolution rate of a drug therefore this parameter can be used to prolong the action of a drug.

3. Viscosity and Nature of the Vehicle

By increasing the viscosity of the vehicle the absorption can be slowed down to a desired extent. Gelatin, carboxymethyl cellulose, polyvinylpyrrolidone and polyvinyl alcohol have been used individually as thickening agents to prolong the action of intramuscular injections. Lipophilic solutions of a drug usually have longer therapeutic effect than the aqueous solutions of the same drug. Therefore oily vehicles may be employed to obtain sustained action of a drug.

Vaso-constriction, immiscibility, dissolution rate, ionization, polymorphism and surface tension of dissolution medium are still other parameters which can prolong the action of a drug.

Types of Sustained-Action Dosage Forms

(a) Long-acting Capsules (Spansules)

The coated beads or granules are filled into hard gelatin capsules which release the medication gradually and uniformly over an extended period of time. They are available in the market under different trade names

(b) Long-acting Multilayer Tablets

In long-acting multilayered tablets the quickly disintegrating portions are compressed successively in the second and third layers. The first layer disintegrates immediately to produce rapid action whereas the other layers disintegrate slowly and continuously to produce prolonged action.

(c) Long-acting Core Tablets

These tablets consists of core tablets containing active medicament or medicaments. The cores are then coated with a substance like glyceryl ester of a higher fatty acid which does not allow the core to disintegrate in the stomach but disinegrates in the intestinal fluids. To this coated core is then applied another coating of active ingredients by means of pan coating. This outer layer disintegrates immediately to produce rapid therapeutic effect there-after the drug is slowly released from the inner core and the patient receives the second dose.

(d) Long-acting Liquid Products

The very finely coated particles of a drug are suspended in a suitable viscous aqueous vehicle to get a suspension.

(e) Repeat-action Tablets

These tablets consists of a core and a coat containing two doses of the medicament. The first dose is compressed or coated in the outer covering whereas the second dose is present in the core. In repeat action tablets the second dose of the drug is released only when the first dose has been completely used up and there is no continuous release of the drug.

Nanocapsules

Nanocapsules, the ultrafine drug delivery system have become very popular due to the reason that they are able to alter the drug distribution. Nanocapsules are quite commonly used for this purpose because they are relatively easy to prepare, pharmaceutically stable and their biodegradation can be controlled. Nanocapsules or nanoparticles are less than a micrometer in dimensions. They consists of a solid or liquid core material containing one or more drugs which are enclosed in coating. The core is known as nucleus or fill whereas coating is known as wall or shell. When a distinct coating and core regions are present then they are known as nanocapsules but when there is no distinct coating and core regions present then they are known as nanoparticles. Materials like gelatin, albumin and casein obtained from natural sources and synthetic substances like diethylacrylates, cyanoacrylates, polyacrylamide etc are used to make nanocapsules or nanoparticles. The drugs which are nanocapsulated include antibiotics, analgesics, steriods, enzymes, toxins, anticancer agents etc.

2. Transdermal Drug Delivery Systems

These systems deliver drugs systamically through the skin but without the use or needle or any other instrument to inject them into the blood circulation. The system is applied to the skin and is absorbed by a process of molecular diffusion. This diffusion process begins as soon the system is applied to the skin. In the begining the process is quite fast till the binding sites of the skin are saturated, then the release of the drug settles at a constant rate.

The drugs to be administered by transdermal route should have the qualities that (1) It should show sufficient absorption through the skin to produce minimum effective concentration (2) It should not produce any harmful effects on the skin on continuous use for a long time. A large number of drugs are already available in the form of transdermal systems and there is a great scope for the further expansion of these systems. The transdermal drug delivery systems has the following advantages :

1. Effects on the liver are eliminated
2. Side effects are reduced
3. Duration of action is increased
4. Patient compliance is improved.

3. Ophthalmic Drug Delivery Systems

The use of conventional opthalmic preparations show lower bioavailability because of constant lacrimal secretion as well as naso-lacrimal drainage. These factors lead to frequent instillation of concentrated preparation into the eyes to obtain the desired therapeutic effects which sometimes leads to undesirable side effects. These difficulties can be overcome by the use of sustained release ophthalmic preparations. The therapeutic effects can be achieved by increasing the contact time between the drug and the corneal surfaces. The sustained action of ophthalmic formulations can be produced (i) by the use of viscous gels and (ii) by the use of some suitable inserts.

4. Contraceptive New Drug Delivery Systems

The new drug delivery systems used for contraception has the following advantages :

1. It eliminates the necessity of administration of the drugs daily.
2. it decreases the systemic or local side effects on the female reproductive systems.
3. It decreases the possible carcinogenic effects of steroids.
4. It allows complete privacy for the women.

The drug delivery systems used as contraceptives can be classified as :

(i) Monthly injections
(ii) Medicated intra-uterine or vaginal devices.
(iii) Implants.

Injections are given to the women which are repeated every month.

Medicated intra-uterine or vaginal devices are quite useful and have certain advantages that they reduce the side effects and possible development of cancer can be minimised or even eliminated. The contraceptive action of these devices can be terminated at any time by removing the device. However these devices has certain disadvantages that they may produce discomfort to the women and menstrual cycle may become irregular. Since intra uterine devices are special devices and require technique for their insertion so a qualified doctor or nurse should insert such type of devices. Copper-T is the most commonly used device of this kind.

Contraceptive implant is a special type of tablet which is kept under the skin by giving a suitable surgical cut which is stiched after inserting the implant. These implants contain levonorgestrel which is continuously released to produce contraceptive action.

2
Pharmacopoeias and Formularies

The books containing the standards for drugs and other related substances are known as pharmacopoeias and formularies, collectively these books are known as the drug compendia. The pharmacopoeias or formularies contain a list of drugs and other related substances regarding their source, descriptions, tests, formulas for preparing the same, action and uses, doses, storage conditions etc. These books are prepared under the authority of the government of the respective countries. The word pharmacopoeia is derived from the Greek words pharmakon means a drug and poieo means make. Literally it means that it is a list of medicinal substances, crude drugs and formulae for making preparations from them.

These books are revised from time to time so as to introduce the latest information available as early as possible after they become established. In order to introduce new products and to keep the size of book within reasonable limits it becomes necessary to omit certain less frequently used drugs and pharmaceutical adjuvants from each new edition of the book. Therefore in each new edition of these books certain new monographs are added while the older ones are deleted.

For the preparation of these books the expert opinion of medical practitioners, teachers and pharmaceutical manufacturers is obtained.

Classification

The drug compendia are classified as :
(i) Official compendia
(ii) Non-official compendia.

(i) Official compendia :

Official compendia are the compilations of drugs and other related substances which are recognised as legal standards of purity, quality and strength by a government agency of respective countries of their origin. Official compendias include British Pharmacopoeia, British Pharmaceutical Codex, Indian Pharmacopoeia, United States Pharmacopoeia, National Formulary, The State Pharmacopoeia of USSR and Pharmacopoeias of other countries.

(ii) Non-official compendia :

The books other than official drug compendia which are used as secondary reference sources for drugs and other related substances are known as non-official drug compendia. These include Merck Index, Remington's Pharmaceutical Sciences, The United States Dispensatory etc.

Official Drug Compendias

1. National Formulary of India

For the compilation of National formulary of India a committee known as national formulary committee was constituted in November 1956 who was assigned the work to compile this formulary. The opinions of medical associations, hospitals, teaching institutions and leading manufacturers in the country were invited and finalised by the committee. it was printed in India by the manager, Government of India Press, Simla in 1960.

2. Pharmacopoeia of India (The Indian Pharmacopoeia)

In 1946 the Government of India published the Indian Pharmacopoeial list which served as a supplement to British

Pharmacopoeia. This list included the drugs which were of substantial medicinal value and were later on included in the Pharmacopoeia. After the publication of this list, the Government of India constituted a permanent Indian Pharmacopoeia Committee in 1948. This committee was assigned the work to prepare Indian Pharmacopoeia and to keep it upto date. The first edition of Indian Pharmacopoeia was published in 1955 and a supplement of it was published in 1960.

The work of revision of the Indian pharmacopoeia as well as the compilation of new edition was taken up simultaneously under the chairmanship of Dr. B.N. Ghosh, Professor of Pharmacology, R.G. Kar, Medical College, Calcutta; who died in 1958. After Dr. B.N. Ghosh, Dr. B. Mukerji Director, Central Drug Research Institute, Lucknow was appointed as chairman of the Indian Pharmacopoeia Committee. The second edition of the Indian Pharmacopoeia was published in 1966 and a supplement of it was published in 1975.

On 30th June 1978, the Indian Pharmacopoeia Committee was reconstituted by the Government of India, Ministry of Health and Family Welfare, under the chairmanship of Dr. Nitya Nand, Director, Central Drug Research Institute, Lucknow. This committee was assigned the work for the preparation of the third edition of the Indian Pharmacopoeia. A working group was constituted by the committee to prepare monographs, appendices and general notes which were finalised by the Pharmacopoeia Committee. The same were published in the form of the Pharmacopoeia of India in 1985, in two volumes, volume I and volume II by the Controller of Publications, Delhi on behalf of Government of India, Ministry of Health and Family Welfare. The volume I contains legal notices, preface, acknowledgements, introduction, general notices and monographs from A to P. The volume II contains monographs from Q to Z, appendices, contents of appendices and index.

For the preparation of Pharmacopoeia of India, the pharmacopoeias of other countries like British, Europe, United States, USSR, Japan, the National Formulary (U.S.A.) and Merck Index were consulted. The persons working in pharmaceutical industry, drug control laboratories, research and teaching institutions also actively participated.

Under the Drugs and Cosmetics Act 1940, the Indian Pharmacopoeia is an official book which contains the standards for drugs and other related substances included in the Pharmacopoeia. The drugs and other related substances prepared by pharmaceutical manufacturers must comply with these standards.

3. British Pharmacopoeia

The responsibility of publishing the British Pharmacopoeia has rested upon the General Medical Council since the Medical Act 1858. The provisions and duties of this council are contained in section 47 of the Medical Act, 1956. According to the recommendations of the Macmillan Committee, the work of preparing new editions of the pharmacopoeia was entrusted by the General Medical Council to the Pharmacopoeia Commission.

The Pharmacopoeia Commission is reconstituted from time to time for a period which corresponds to the period during which a new edition of the British Pharmacopoeia is prepared and published. Since 1948 the new edition of British Pharmacopoeia is published at intervals of five years i.e. 1948, 1953, 1958, 1963, 1968, 1973. After 1973 the new edition was published in 1980 and then in 1988. In addition to the publication of the pharmacopoeia, the addendums are also published from time to time in between two main editions.

The British Pharmacopoeia 1980, the thirteenth edition and 1988, the fourteenth edition was published by Her Majesty's Stationery Office for the Health Ministers on the recommendations of the Medicines Commission in accordance with the Medicines Act 1968.

British Pharmacopoeia is the source of official standards for drugs in the United Kingdom and other parts of the world. Generations of pharmaceutical students were brought up to regard the pharmacopoeia as the main source of all their pharmaceutical knowledge. Now a days the pharmacopoeia also provides knowledge about pharmaceutical products regarding standards and methods of analysis to be employed.

4. British Pharmaceutical Codex

It was in 1903 that the Council of the Pharmaceutical Society of Great Britain decided to prepare a reference book for the use of medical practitioners and dispensing pharmacists. The first edition of the British Pharmaceutical Codex was published in 1907. The subsequent revisions of this codex were published in 1911, 1923, 1934, 1949, 1954, 1959, 1963, 1968, 1973.

On the request of British Pharmacopoeia Commission, the Council of the Pharmaceutical Society agreed in 1959 for the publication of Codex to coincide with that of the British Pharmacopoeia, so that these two books i.e. British Pharmaceutical Codex and British Pharmacopoeia should come into effect on the same dates.

The British Pharmaceutical Codex differs from British Pharmacopoeia in that :

(a) It contains many more drugs and preparations; some may be included in advance of the pharmacopoeia and may acquire the official status while other drugs may have been included in the former editions of Pharmacopoeia but now they are retained in the Codex because they are still commonly used.

(b) It provides standards for drugs, surgical dressings and pharmaceutical preparations not included in the British Pharmacopoeia.

(c) It provides information on the actions and uses of drugs, their undesirable effects, precautions and the treatment of poisoning.

(d) It contains formulae, method of preparation, dose, container and storage conditions of most of the preparations which are still extemporaneously prepared in the pharmacy and dispensed by the pharmacists. These preparations include mixtures, powders, eye drops, ear drops, liniments, lotions, ointments, creams, pastes, suppositories etc.

5. The United States Pharmacopoeia

The United States Pharmacopoeia and the National Formulary (USP-NF) are recognised as official compendia and are used as reference books for determining the strength, quality, purity, packaging and labelling of drugs and other related articles.

The United States Pharmacopoeia was originally published in 1820 under the authority of the United States Pharmacopoeial Convention and the National Formulary was published in 1888 under the guidance of the American Pharmaceutical Association. In 1974 the National Formulary was purchased by the United States Pharmacopoeial Convention and from 1980 onwards only one official book of drug standards was published under the heading, The United States Pharmacopoeia and The National Formulary (USP-NF).

6. Extra Pharmacopoeia (Martindale)

The Extra Pharmacopoeia was first produced in 1883 by William Martindale and is still known as "Martindale". This is an authorised reference book on drugs and is used throughout the world. It provides all sorts of latest information on drugs and medicines. The Extra Pharmacopoeia is prepared by consulting the pharmacopoeias of other countries. The twenty eighth edition was published in December 1982. The twentyninth edition was published in January 1989 by direction of the Council of the Royal Pharmaceutical Society of Great Britain and prepared in the society's Department of Pharmaceutical Sciences.

7. The Merck Index

It is an encyclopedia of chemicals, drugs and biologicals. The first edition was published in 1889 and the eleventh edition was published in 1989 by Merck & Co; Inc. Rahway. N.J., U.S.A.

8. The International Pharmacopoeia

The International Pharmacopoeia is published by the World Health Organisation and is particularly used in developing countries.

9. State Pharmacopoeia of the USSR

The first edition of the State Pharmacopoeia of the Union of Soviet Socialist Republics was published in 1866 in Russian language. It was followed by next editions in 1871, 1880, 1891, 1902, 1910, 1925, 1946, 1961 so on. The 9th edition was published in 1961 under the auspices of the Pharmacopoeia Committee of the Ministry of Health of the USSR. Research institutes, pharmaceutical teaching institutions, industrial houses and specialists of highest qualifications were actively associated with the publication of the pharmacopoeias.

Other useful Books and Periodicals :

Textbooks

1. Bentley's Textbook of Pharmaceutics by H. Davis.
2. Remington's Pharmaceutical Sciences, Mack Publishing Company, Pennsylvania.
3. Introduction to Pharmaceutical Dosage Forms by H.C. Ansel (Lea and Febiger)
4. Dispensing of Medication by E.W. Martin; Mack Publishing Co,
5. Dispensing for pharmaceutical students by Cooper and Gunn; Pitman Publishing Company, London.
6. The Theory and Practice of Industrial Pharmacy by Leon Lachman published by Varghese Publishing House, Hind Rajasthan Building, Dadar, Bombay. 400014.

Journals

1. *Indian Journal of Pharmaceutical Sciences :*
   It is a scientific publication of the Indian Pharmaceutical Association. It was formerly known as the Indian Journal of Pharmacy.

2. *Indian Journal of Pharmaceutical Education :*
   This journal is the official publication of Association of Pharmaceutical Teachers of India and is published quarterly in March, June, September and December every year.

3. *The Eastern Pharmacist :*

   It is published on the 15th day of every month from New Delhi located at 507, Ashok Bhawan, 93 Nehru Place, New Delhi-110016 and published on behalf of the Eastern Pharmacist from E-38, Hauz Khas, New Delhi-110016

4. *American Journal of Pharmaceutical Education :*

   It is the official publication of American Association of Colleges of Pharmacy. Its purpose is to document pharmaceutical education and to advance it.

5. *Journal of Medicinal Chemistry :*

   It is published biweekly by the American Chemical Society at 1155 16th St. N.W. Washington DC 20036.

6. *Pharma Today :*

   It is a monthly pharmaceutical trade magazine edited and published by G.S. Rao on behalf of Sharavathi Management Services, C5/19-24, Sector 3, P.O. Konkan Bhawan, C.B.D; New Bombay-400614

3
Weights and Measures

Weight :

It is a measure of the gravitational force acting on a body and is directly proportional to its mass. The mass remains constant and never varies because it is based on inertia whereas weight varies slightly with change in latitude, altitude, temperature and pressure. The effect of these factors is not considered unless very accurate weighings are to be done.

Measure :

It is the measurement of volume of any substance. Temperature and pressure exert their effect specially on liquids and gases. The effect of these factors is only taken into consideration when accurate preparations are to be made.

There are two systems of weights and measures (a) the imperial system (b) the metric system, with which the pharmacist must be familiar. The imperial system is an old system based on arbitrary and unrelated units e.g. grains, drachms, ounces and gallons whereas the metric system or decimal system is based on related and rationally derived units e.g. milligrams, grams, centimeters, meters, millilitres, litres etc. Because of its easier calculations, greater accuracy and flexibility and use in other sciences, now a days this is the most widely used system by official agencies.

In 1948 a committee on weights and measures legislation was appointed by the president of the Board of Trade to review the existing weights and measures legislation and to make recommendations thereof. In 1951 the committee published a report in which it was recommended that the apothecary system (Imperial system) should be abolished and the metric system should be adopted in its place. Therefore steps were taken to abolish the use of imperial system for all dealings in drugs and medicines and its use was declared illegal in pharmacy profession. Since 31st March 1969 pharmacists were required to carry out all dispensing work in metric system.

Accordingly the first change over to the metric system appeared in the British Pharmacopoeia and British Pharmaceutical Codex published in 1963. The doses of tablets, capsules and injections were given only in metric quantities. Weights and Measures Regulations 1964 described certain equivalents in metric units that whenever strength is prescribed in the imperial units that must be dispensed according to equivalent strength in metric units.

Though the pharmacists are required to use the metric system for dispensing the prescriptions but still a large number of physicians trained to use the imperial system prescribe the drugs in the old system and some hospitals still retain it as the local standard. Some drugs are prescribed in fractional doses (1/200, 1/150, 1/100 gr.). The bottles for liquids are still manufactured to contain ounce measurements rather than milliliters.

Due to the above mentioned reasons, it is still necessary to be familiar with both the systems which are described in detail as follows :

(a) Imperial system

Imperial system is divided into two systems.

(i) Avoirdupois system

(ii) Apothecaries system.

Avoirdupois system

According to this system the standard unit for weighing is pound and all other measures of mass are derived from pound. It is represented by lb.

1 lb = 16 oz (avoir)

1 lb = 7000 grains

1 lb = 7000/16 437.5 grains

Apothecaries system:

It is known as troy system. The standard weight in this system is grain.

20 grain	=	1 scruple
60 grain	=	1 drachm
480 grain	=	1 ounce (Apothe)
8 drachm	=	1 ounce (Apothe)
12 ounces (Apothe)	=	1 pound (Apothe)
5760 grain	=	1 pound (Apothe)

Abbreviations commonly used in weighing

Latin name	Symbol	English Name	Equal to
Granum	gr	grain	1 grain
Scrupulus	℈	Scruple	20 grain
Drachma	ʒ	drachm	60 grain
Uncia	oz	ounce (Avoir)	437.5 grain
Uncia	℥	ounce (Apothe)	480 grains
Libra	lb	pound (Avoir)	7000 grains
Libra	lb	pound (Apothe)	5760 grains

Measures of Capacity

Standard units for capacity are same in avoirdupois as well as apothecaries system. The standard unit is gallon and all other measures of capacity are derived from gallon.

1 gallon	= 160 fluid ounces.	
1/4th of a gallon	= 1 quart	= 40 fl. ounce.
1/8th of a gallon	= 1 pint	= 20 fl. ounce.
1/60th of a gallon	= 1 fl. ounce.	
1/8th of one fl. ounce	= 1 fl. drachm.	
1/60th of one fl. drachm	= 1 minim.	
1 fluid ounce	= 480 minim.	
1 fluid drachm	= 480/8	= 60 minim.

Abbreviations Commonly Used in Measures of Capacity

Latin name	Symbol	English name	Equal to
Minimum	m	minim	1 minim
Fluidrachma	ʒ	fl. drachm	60 minim

Fluidunicia	℥	fl. ounce	480 minim
Octarius	O	pint	20 fl. ounces
Congius	C	gallon	160 fl. ounces

Metric System

Standard unit of measures of mass (weight) is kilogram and all other measures of mass are derived from kilogram

1 Kilogram (kg)	= 1000 gm	
1 Hectogram (hg)	= 100 gm	
1 Decagram (dag)	= 10 gm	
1 Gram (gm)	= 1 gm	
1 Decigram (dg)	= 0.1 gm	= 100 mg
1 Centigram (cg)	= 0.01 gm	= 10 mg
1 Milligram (mg)	= 0.001 gm	= 1 mg
1 Microgram (μg, mcg)		= 1/1000 mg

Measures of Capacity

Standard unit for measures of capacity (volume) is litre and all other measures of capacity are derived from litre.

1 litre (lt) = 1000 millilitre (ml)

Domestic Measures :

1 drop	= 1 minim = 0.06 ml	
1 tea spoonful	= 1 fl. drachm	= 4 ml
1 desert spoonful	= 2 fl. drachm	= 8 ml
1 table spoonful	= 4 fl. drachm	= 15 ml
2 table spoonful	= 1 fl. ounce	= 30 ml
1 wine glassful	= 2 fl. ounce	= 60 ml
1 tea cupful = 4 fl. ounce	= 120 ml	
1 tumblerful	= 8 fl. ounce	= 240 ml

Conversion Factors :

1 grain	= 64.8 mg	= 65 mg (for all practical purposes)	
1 drop	= 1 minim	= 0.06 ml	-do-
1 fl. ounce	= 29.57 ml	= 30 ml	-do-
1 gram	= 15.43 gr	= 15 gr	-do-
1 milligram	= 1/65 gr	= 1/65 gr	-do-

1 millilitre = 16.23 minim = 15 m -do-
1 litre = 33.8 fl. ounce
1 kilogram = 2.2 pound

3.1 Calculations :

Calculations based on density :

Density in defined as the mass of a substance per unit volume. It has the units of mass over volume.

Specific gravity is the ratio of the weight of a substance in air to that of an equal volume of water. It does not have any units.

In the metric system both density and specific gravity are numerically equal. The density, weight and volume of any substance can be calculated from the following equations :

$$\text{Density} = \frac{\text{weight}}{\text{volume}}$$

$$\text{Weight} = \text{density} \times \text{volume}$$

$$\text{Volume} = \frac{\text{weight}}{\text{density}}$$

If any two variables are given, the third one can be calculated.

1. Calculate the weight of 120 ml of an oil whose density is 0.9624 gm/ml

$$\text{Weight} = \text{density} \times \text{volume}$$
$$= 0.9624 \text{ gm/ml} \times 120 \text{ ml}$$
$$= 115.488 \text{ gm}$$

2. Calculate the volume of 200 gm of glycerin. The density of glycerin is 1.25 gm/ml

$$\text{Volume} = \frac{\text{weight}}{\text{density}}$$
$$= \frac{200 \text{ gm}}{1.2 \text{ gm/ml}} = 166.6 \text{ ml}$$

3. Calculate the weight of 1 litre of alcohol whose density is 0.816 gm/ml

$$\text{Weight} = \text{density} \times \text{volume}$$
$$= 0.816 \text{ gm/ml} \times 1000 \text{ ml}$$
$$= 816 \text{ gm}$$

Conversions from Imperial to metric and metric to Imperial systems.

1. How many mg are in one grain

$$\text{Since } 15.43 \text{ gr} = 1.0 \text{ gm}$$

$$1 \text{ gr} = \frac{1.000}{15.43} \text{ gm} = 0.0648 \text{ gm}$$

$$= 64.8 \text{ mg}$$

$$\therefore 1 \text{ gr} = 64.8 \text{ mg}$$

2. How many grams are in 1 ounce (Apoth)

$$1 \text{ ounce (Approx)} = 480 \text{ gr}$$

$$\text{Since } 15.43 \text{ gr} = 1.00 \text{ gm}$$

$$1 \text{ gr} = \frac{1.000}{15.43}$$

$$480 \text{ gr} = \frac{1.000}{15.43} \times 480 = 31.11 \text{ gm}$$

$$\therefore 1 \text{ ounce (Apoth)} = 31.11 \text{ gm}$$

3. How many grams are in 1 ounce (Avoir)

$$1 \text{ ounce (Avoir)} = 437.5 \text{ gr}$$

$$\text{Since } 15.43 \text{ gr} = 1.000 \text{ gm}$$

$$1 \text{ gr} = \frac{1.000}{15.43} \text{ gm}$$

$$437.5 \text{ gr} = \frac{1.000}{15.43} \times 437.5 = 28.35 \text{ gm}$$

$$\therefore 1 \text{ ounce (Avoir)} = 28.35 \text{ gr}$$

4. How many ml are in 1 fl oz

$$1 \text{ fl.oz} = 480 \text{ m}$$

$$16.23 \text{ m} = 1 \text{ ml}$$

$$1 \text{ m} = \frac{1}{16.23}$$

$$480 \text{ m} = \frac{1}{16.23} \times 480 = 29.57 \text{ ml}$$

$$\therefore 1 \text{ fl.oz} = 29.57 \text{ ml}$$

5. Convert 3 drachm into mgs

$$1 \text{ drachm} = 60 \text{ gr}$$

$$3 \text{ drachm} = 60 \times 3 = 180 \text{ gr}$$

$$1 \text{ gr} = 64.8 \text{ mg}$$

$$180 \text{ gr} = 64.8 \times 180 = 11664 \text{ mg}$$
$$\therefore 3 \text{ dhrachm} = 11664 \text{ mg}$$

6. Convert 550 mg into grains

$$1 \text{ mg} = \frac{1}{64.8} \text{ gr}$$
$$550 \text{ mg} = \frac{1}{64.8} \times 550 = 8.48 \text{gr}$$

7. Convert $\frac{1}{100}$gr into metric weights

$$1 \text{ gr} = 64.8 \text{ mg}$$
$$\frac{1}{100} \text{ gr} = 64.8 \times \frac{1}{100} = .648 \text{ mg}$$

8. Convert $\frac{1}{6}$ gr into mgs

$$1 \text{ gr} = 64.8 \text{ mg}$$
$$\frac{1}{6} \text{ gr} = 64.8 \times \frac{1}{6} = 10.8 \text{ mg}$$

9. Convert 30 m into ml

$$16.23 \text{ m} = 1 \text{ ml}$$
$$1 \text{ m} = \frac{1}{16.23} \text{ ml}$$
$$30 \text{ m} = \frac{1}{16.23} \times 30 = 1.848 \text{ ml}$$

10. Convert 2 pt into ml

$$1 \text{ pt} = 20 \text{ fl.oz}$$
$$2 \text{ pt} = 20 \times 2 = 40 \text{ fl.oz}$$
$$1 \text{ fl.oz} = 29.57 \text{ ml}$$
$$40 \text{ fl.oz} = 29.57 \times 40 = 1182.8 \text{ ml}$$
$$\therefore 2 \text{ pt} = 1182.8 \text{ ml}$$

3.2 Calculations based on Imperial systems :

For preparing 1% w/v solns any of the following formulas which are identical in strength can be used :

	I	II	III	IV
Solid	1 gr	4.375 gr	35 gr	1 oz (Avoir)
Solvent to produce	110 m	1 fl.oz	8 fl.oz	100 fl.oz

Formula I should be used when the volume of the solution required is small and the strength of such solution is weak. Formula II, III & IV may be used according to the quantities of the solutions to be prepared.

While using formula I it is important to note that it is not permitted to weigh less than 1 gr of solid on the dispensing balance because of its low sensitivity hence the volume prepared may be much more than the required volume. The excess volume so prepared may be rejected or preserved for further prescriptions to be dispensed.

1. Rx

Atropine sulphate	1/2%
Aqua q.s.	ʒ ii

Calculations :

1 gr of Atropine sulphate dissolved in 110 m = 1% W/V soln

1 gr of Atropine sulphate dissolved in 220 m = 1/2% W/V soln

Dispense 120 m or 2 drachms out of the above soln and reject the remainder.

2. Prepare 1 oz of 1/8% solution of zinc sulphate in equal volumes of normal saline solution and Adrenaline solution.

Calculations :

Since two solvents i.e. normal saline solution and Adrenaline solution are used out of which Adrenaline solution is costlier than normal saline solution therefore dissolve zinc sulphate at double strength in normal saline solution.

1 gr of zinc sulphate dissolved in 110 m of normal saline solution = 1% W/V soln

1 gr of zinc sulphate dissolved in 440 m of normal saline solution = 1/4% W/V soln

Take out 240 m of the above solution and mix it with 240 m of Adrenaline solution. The resulting 480 m (1 oz) solution will be 1/8%

3. Prepare 4 oz of a 5% solution of a substance.

Calculations :

35 gr dissolved in 8 fl. oz = 1% W/V soln

35 x 5 gr dissolved in 8 fl. oz = 5% W/V soln

$\frac{35 \times 5}{8}$ gr dissolved in one fl oz = 5% W/V soln

$\frac{35 \times 5 \times 4}{8}$ gr dissolved in 4 fl oz = 5% W/V soln

= 87.5 gr

∴ weigh 87.5 gr of the substance and dissolve in sufficient amount of water to produce 4 fl. oz. The resulting solution will be 5% solution

4. Send 1 pint of a 1 in 500 solution of Potassium permanganate.

Calculations :

35 gr of Potassium permanganate dissolved in 8 fl. oz = 1% W/V soln

$35 \times \frac{100}{500}$ gr of Potassium permanganate dissolved in 8 fl. oz $= \frac{1}{5}$% W/V soln (1 in 500)

$\frac{35 \times 100}{500 \times 8}$ gr of Potassium permanganate dissolved in one fl. oz $= \frac{1}{5}$% W/V soln

$\frac{35 \times 100 \times 20}{500 \times 8}$ gr of Potassium permanganate dissolved in 20 fl.oz $= \frac{1}{5}$% W/V soln

= 17.5 gr

Therefore weigh 17.5 gr of Pot. permanganate and dissolve in sufficient amount of water to produce 1 pint. The resulting solution will be 1 in 500 solution.

5. How many tablets each containing 8.75 gr of Mercuric chloride will be required to make one quart of 0.05 % solution.

Calculations :

35 gr dissolved in 8 fl. oz = 1% W/V soln.

35×0.05 gr dissolved in 8 fl. oz = 0.05% W/V soln

$\frac{35 \times 0.05}{8}$ gr dissolved in one fl. oz = 0.05% W/V soln

$\frac{35 \times 0.05}{8} \times 40$ gr dissolved in 40 fl. oz = 0.05% W/V soln

$= \frac{35 \times 5 \times 40}{8 \times 100} = 8.75$ gr

8.75 gr of mercuric chloride are contained in = 1 tablet

1 gr of mercuric chloride are contained in = $\frac{1}{8.75}$

8.75 gr of mercuric chloride will be

contained in $= \frac{1}{8.75} \times 8.75$

= 1 tablet

Therefore each tablet of 8.75 gr of Mercuric chloride will make one quart of 0.05% solution.

Solutions dispensed in concentrated form :

6. Required 6 oz of a solution so that 2 teaspoonfuls diluted to a pint will make a 1 in 1000 solution.
This problem will be solved in two parts.

(a) Calculate the no of grains required to make one pint of a 1 in 1000 solution

(b) Every two teaspoonfuls of the concentrated solution must contain these number of grains. Therefore multiply these number of grains with the number of two teaspoonfuls contained in 6 oz.

(a) 35 gr dissolved in 8 fl oz = 1 in 100 soln

$\frac{35 \times 100}{1000}$ gr dissolved in 8 fl. oz = 1 in 1000 soln

$\frac{35 \times 100}{1000 \times 8}$ gr dissolved in one fl. oz = 1 in 1000 soln

$\frac{35 \times 100 \times 20}{1000 \times 8}$ gr dissolved in 20 fl. oz = 1 in 1000 soln

= 8.75 gr

∴ 8.75 gr of the drug must be contained in every 2 teaspoonfuls of the solution.

(b) 6 oz = 6 × 8 = 48 teaspoonfuls

2 teaspoonfuls contain = 8.75 gr

1 teaspoonful contains = $\frac{8.75}{2}$ gr

48 teaspoonfuls must contain = $\frac{8.75}{2} \times 48 = 210$gr

∴ Dissolve 210 gr of the drug in water and dilute to 6 fl oz.

Sometimes concentrated solutions may be prescribed and the pharmacist is asked to label with directions to prepare weaker percentage solutions.

7. Send 4 oz of a 10% solution of Potassium permanganate and label with directions for preparing a quart of a 1 in 400 solution.

Calculations :

These types of problems are also calculated in two parts

(a) Calculate the number of grains required to make 4 oz of a 10% solution

(b) Calculate the quantity to be diluted to a quart to make a 1 in 400 solution.

(a) 35 gr dissolved in 8 fl. oz = 1% W/V soln

35 × 10 gr dissolved in 8 fl oz = 10% W/V soln

$\frac{35 \times 10}{8}$ gr dissolved in one fl. oz = 10% W/V soln

$\frac{35 \times 10 \times 4}{8}$ gr dissolved in 4 fl. oz = 10% W/V soln

= 175 gr

∴ Dissolve 175 gr in water and dilute it to 4 fl oz.

(b) A 10% solution means 1 in $\frac{100}{10}$ = 1 in 10 soln

That is 10 oz of the solution contains 1 oz of the substance

∴ 10 oz of this solution diluted to 400 oz will produce 1 in 400 solution.

$$\therefore \frac{10 \times 40}{400} = 1 \text{ oz diluted to one quart will produce 1 in}$$

400 solution.

Therefore label with directions to dilute 1 oz or 2 tablespoonfuls to a quart

3.3 Exercises (A)

Calculate the quantities required to prepare the following :

1. Atropine sulphate 1% send 4 drachms
2. Acriflavine 0.1% in a mixture of equal volume of alcohol and water, send 2 oz.
3. 8 oz of a 1 in 2000 solution
4. 1 gallon of a 1 in 1000 solution
5. 1 pint of a 0.01% solution
6. 4 oz of a 0.625% solution
7. 1 quart of a normal suline solution
8. How many tablets each containing 8.75 gr of corrosive sublimate will be required to make 1 pint of a 0.4% solution.
9. 8 oz of a solution so that 1 tablespoonful to half a gallon makes 1 in 500 solution
10. 8 oz so that 1 tablespoonful to half a gallon will make a 1 in 2000 solution
11. 10 oz of a 2.5% solution and label with the directions for preparing a quart of 0.0625% solution.
12. 10 oz of 6% solution and label with the directions for preparing 30 oz of a 0.05% solution.
13. From 20% solution supplied prepare a quart of a 0.0625% solution
14. From 8% solution supplied prepare 1 pint of a 1 in 1000 solution.

3.4 Calculations based on metric system

1. Calculate the formula for 40 gm coaltar and zinc ointment from the official formula given below :

Yellow soft paraffin	600 gm
Zinc oxide, finely sifted	300 gm
Strong coaltar solution	100 gm

$$\text{quantities required for 40 gm} = \frac{40}{1000} \times \text{official quantities.}$$

2. Calculate the formula for 250 ml of oily lotion of calamine from the formula given below :

Calamine	50 gm
Wool fat	10 gm
Oleic acid	5 ml
Arachis oil	500 ml
Calcium hydroxide solution sufficient to produce	1000 ml

$$\text{Quantities required for 250 ml} = \frac{250}{1000} \times \text{ quantities given.}$$

3. Rx

Hyoscine hydrobromide 0.6 mg

Make powders. Send such 10 powders.

Calculations :

To get the required quantities for 10 powders, multiply the given quantity by 10.

4. Rx

Heavy magnesium carbonate	8.125 gm
Light magnesium carbonate	8.125 gm
Rhubarb, in powder	6.25 gm
Ginger, in powder	2.5 gm

Make powder. Send 100 gm.

Calculations :

To get the required quantities for 100 gm, multiply the given quantities by 4.

Percentage Calculations

(i) *Weight in Volume (W/V) Solutions*

In this the solute is weighed and the solvent is measured. The general formula for 1% W/V solution is :

Solid	1 part by weight
Solvent to produce	100 parts by volume.

1 gm solute dissolved in sufficient amount of water to produce 100 ml or 10 mg in 1 ml of water make 1% W/V solution. Unless and until specially specified the solutions in pharmacy are supplied as W/V solutions.

(ii) *Weight in Weight (W/W) Solutions*

In this the solute and the solvent are taken be weight. The general formula for 1% W/W solution is :

Solid	1 part by weight
Solvent to produce	100 parts by weight.

Percentage solutions of solids in liquids are not made W/W unless specially requested.

(iii) *Volume by Volume (V/V) Solutions*

In this the solute and the solvent are taken by volume. The general formula for 1% V/V solution is :

Solute	1 part by volume
Solvent to produce	100 parts by volume

1 ml solute dissolved in sufficient amount of solvent to produce 100 ml.

5. Calculate the quantity of sodium chloride required to prepare 500 ml of a 2% solution.

Calculations :

1 gm of sodium chloride dissolved in water to produce 100 ml = 1% W/V soln.

1 x 2 gm of sodium chloride dissolved in water to produce 100 ml =2% W/V soln.

For 500 ml the quantity of sodium chloride required

$$= \frac{1 \times 2 \times 500}{100} = 10 \text{ gm.}$$

Therefore dissolve 10 gm of sodium chloride in sufficient amount of water to produce 500 ml. The resulting solution will be 2% solution.

6. Calculate the quantity of sodium chloride required for preparing 200 ml of a 0.9% solution

Calculations :

1 gm of sodium chloride dissolved in water to produce 100 ml = 1% W/V soln.

1 x 0.9 gm of sodium chloride dissolved in water to produce 100 ml = 0.9% W/V soln.

for 200 ml the quantity of sodium chloride required

$$= \frac{1 \times 0.9 \times 200}{100} = 1.8 \text{ gm.}$$

Therefore dissolve 1.8 gm of sodium chloride in sufficient amount of water to produce 200 ml. The resulting solution will be 0.9% solution.

7. Prepare 30 ml of 10% solution of methyl salicylate in alcohol.

Calculations :

For 100 ml solution the quantity of methyl salicylate required = 10 ml

For 30 ml solution the quantity of methyl salicylate required

$$= \frac{10 \times 30}{100} = 3 \text{ ml.}$$

Therefore mix 3 ml of methyl salicylate with sufficient alcohol to produce 30 ml. The resulting solution will be 10% solution.

8. Prepare 50 ml of 0.1% solution of acriflavine in a mixture of equal volume of alcohol and water.

Calculations :

Alcohol is relatively expensive but water is inexpensive, therefore prepare the acriflavine solution at double strength in water and then add alcohol.

Double the strength of 0.1% = 0.2%

1 gm of acriflavine dissolved in 100 ml of water = 1% W/V soln.

1 x 0.2 gm of acriflavine dissolved in 100 ml of water = 0.2% W/V soln.

for 50 ml solution the quantity of acriflavine required

$$= \frac{1 \times 0.2 \times 50}{100} = 0.1 \text{ gm} = 100 \text{ mg}$$

Therefore dissolve 100 mg of acriflavine in 50 ml water. Out of this measure 25 ml and mix it with 25 ml alcohol. The resulting solution will be 0.1% solution of acriflavine in a mixture of equal volume of alcohol and water.

9. Prepare 100 ml of a 1 in 4000 solution of potassium permanganate.

Calculations :

$$1 \text{ in } 4000 = \frac{100}{4000} \text{ per cent} = 0.025\%$$

1 gm of potassium permanganate dissolved in 100 ml water = 1% W/V soln.

1 x 0.025 gm of potassium permanganate dissolved in 100 ml water = 0.025% W/V soln.

For 100 ml solution the quantity of potassium permanganate required

$$= \frac{1 \times 0.025 \times 100}{100} = 0.025 \text{ gm} = 25 \text{ mg}$$

Therefore dissolve 25 mg of potassium permanganate in sufficient water to produce 100 ml. The resulting solution will be 1 in 4000 solution.

10. Send 150 ml of 4% potassium permanganate solution and label with directions for preparing 500 ml of a 1 in 2500 solution.

Calculations :

(a) 1 gm of potassium permanganate dissolved in 100 ml water = 1% W/V soln.

1 x 4 gm of potassium permanganate dissolved in 100 ml water = 4% W/V soln.

For 150 ml the quantity of potassium permanganate required

$$= \frac{1 \times 4 \times 150}{100} = 6 \text{ gm}$$

Therefore dissolve 6 gm of potassium permanganate in sufficient water to produce 150 ml solution.

(b) Strength of concentrated solution = 4%

Strength of dilute solution = 1 in 2500

$$= \frac{100}{2500} = \frac{1}{25} = 0.04\%$$

$$\text{Degree of dilution} = \frac{4}{0.04} = 100 \text{ times}$$

Quantity of concentrated solution required

$$= \frac{500}{100} = 5 \text{ ml}$$

Therefore dilute 5 ml of concentrated potassium permanganate soln upto 500 ml with water, the resulting solution will be 1 in 2500 solution.

11. From 1 in 400 solution of acriflavine, prepare 100 ml of a 1 in 5000 solution

Calculations :

Strength of concentrated acriflavine soln provided

$$= 1 \text{ in } 400 = \frac{100}{400} = \frac{1}{4} = 0.25\%$$

Strength of dilute solution

$$= 1 \text{ in } 5000 = \frac{100}{5000} = \frac{1}{50} = 0.02\%$$

$$\text{Degree of dilution} = \frac{0.25}{0.02} = \frac{25}{2} \text{ times}$$

Quantity of concentrated solution required

$$= \frac{100 \times 2}{25} = 8 \text{ ml}$$

Therefore dilute 8 ml of concentrated solution of acriflavine upto 100 ml with water, the resulting solution will be 1 in 5000 solution.

Alcohol Dilutions

Dilute alcohols are made from 95% alcohol which contains 95 parts ethyl alcohol and 5 parts water. All other dilutions of alcohol are prepared by mixing the specified parts of alcohol and water.

On mixing alcohol with water, contraction in volume and rise in temperature occurs and mixture becomes turbid. The turbidity is caused by minute air bubbles evolved from the alcohol on dilution, because air is less soluble in water than in alcohol, so on addition of water air is partly expelled from the solution. Since there will be contraction in volume and rise in temperature, consequently it is necessary to cool the mixture to about 20°C before adjusting to the final volume.

The general formula for calculating the amount of stronger alcohol required to make a weaker alcohol is as under :

$$\frac{\textbf{Volume required} \times \textbf{precentage required}}{\textbf{percentage used}} = \textbf{volume of stronger alcohol to be used.}$$

12. Prepare 600 ml of 60% alcohol from 95% alcohol.

Calculations :

Volume of 95% alcohol to be used

$$= \frac{600 \times 60}{95} = 379 \text{ ml}$$

Therefore take 379 ml of 95% alcohol, dilute it upto 600 ml with water, the resulting dilution will contain 60% alcohol.

13. Prepare 500 ml of 40% alcohol from 95% alcohol.

Volume of 95% alcohol to be used

$$= \frac{500 \times 40}{95} = 210 \text{ ml}$$

Therefore dilute 210 ml of 95% alcohol upto 500 ml with water. The resulting dilution will contain 40% alcohol.

Weight in Weight (W/W) Solutions

The general formula is as under :

$$\frac{\textbf{Weight required} \times \textbf{percentage required}}{\textbf{percentage used}} = \textbf{weight of stronger acid to be used.}$$

14. Send 200 ml of a solution of acetic acid containing 4% of real acetic acid. The strength of real acetic acid is 33%

Calculations :

Weight of stronger acid to be used

$$= \frac{200 \times 4}{33} = 24.2 \text{ gm}$$

Therefore weigh 24.2 gm of real acetic acid and dilute it upto 200 ml with water, the resulting solution will contain 4% acetic acid.

15. Send 200 ml of a solution of ammonia containing 4% by weight of ammonia. The strong solution of ammonia contains 32.5% of ammonia W/W

Calculations :

The weight of strong ammonia required

$$= \frac{200 \times 4}{32.5} = 24.615 \text{ gm}$$

Therefore dilute 24.615 gm of strong solution of ammonia to 200 gm with water. The resulting solution will contain 4% ammonia.

3.5 Alligation Method

The calculations for exercises from 12 to 15 may be done by a method known as alligation method. This method is not recommended except as a method of checking because there are chances of errors in writing the figures.

16. Prepare 1000 gm of dilute acetic acid 4% from 33% real acetic acid.

Calculations :

The weight of real acetic acid required

$$= \frac{1000 \times 4}{33} = 121.2 \text{ gm}$$

The amount of water required

$$= 1000 - 121.2 = 878.8 \text{ gm}$$

By Alligation Method

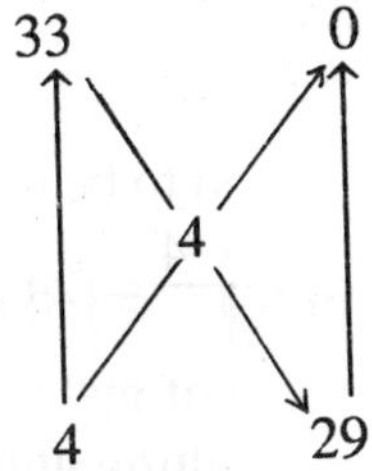

Subtract 0 (for water) from 4 $= 4$

Subtract 4 from 33 $= 29$

4 parts of real acetic acid and 29 parts of water will constitute 33 parts by weight of dilute acetic acid.

Therefore the quantity of real acetic acid required

$$= \frac{1000 \times 4}{33} = 121.2 \text{ gm}$$

and the quantity of water required

$$= \frac{1000 \times 29}{33} = 878.8 \text{ gm}$$

17. Prepare 400 ml of 70% alcohol from 95% alcohol.

Calculations :

Volume of 95% alcohol to be used

$$= \frac{400 \times 70}{95} = 294.74 \text{ ml}$$

Volume of water to be used

$$= 400 - 294 = 103{,}26 \text{ ml}$$

Alligation Method

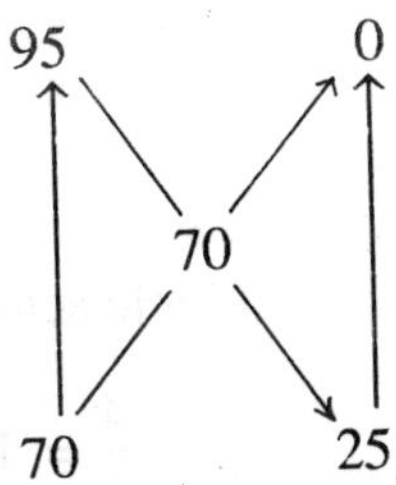

$\therefore$ Quantity of 95% alcohol required

$$= \frac{400 \times 70}{95} = 294.74 \text{ ml}$$

and the quantity of water required

$$= \frac{400 \times 25}{95} = 105.26 \text{ ml}$$

3.6 Exercises (B)

1. Prepare 500 ml of 1 in 5000 solution of Potassium permanganate.
2. Send 100 ml of 2% Acriflavine solution.
3. Supply 500 ml of Normal saline solution.
4. Prepare 300 ml of 45% alcohol from 90% alcohol
5. Prepare 400 ml of 55% alcohol from 95% alcohol.
6. Send 200 ml of 60% alcohol from 95% alcohol.
7. Supply 500 ml of 20% alcohol from 95% alcohol
8. From 90% alcohol provided supply 400 ml of 60% alcohol.
9. From 60% alcohol supplied prepare 2 litres of 45% alcohol.
10. Supply 250 ml of solution containing 15% of Real Acetic acid. The strength of Official Acetic acid is 33.
11. Prepare 120 ml of solution containing 20% of Real Acetic acid. The Real Acetic acid is 33% W/W
12. Prepare 1000 gm of 6% Acetic acid from 33% Acetic acid.

3.7 Isotonic Solutions

All the ophthalmic and injectable solutions should be isotonic e.g. ophthalmic solutions should be isotonic with Lachrymal secretions (tears) to prevent irritation and pain, similarly, injectable solutions should be isotonic with blood plasma. Solutions having the same osmotic pressure are said to be isotonic. As compared to blood plasma if a solution has lower osmotic pressure it is said to be hypotonic but if it has higher osmotic pressure it is said to be hypertonic.

The solutions which are not isotonic with plasma may be harmful to use. On injecting the hypotonic solutions into blood stream, it may enter the red blood cells in an attempt to produce equilibrium. the cells swells rapidly until they burst leading to haemolysis. As this damage is irreversible may lead to serious danger to red blood cells.

When hypertonic solution is injected into the blood stream, the water comes out of the membrane of red blood cells in order to reach equilibrium. The cells shrink leading to crenulation which is only a temporary damage. When the osmotic pressure of two solutions becomes equal the damaged cells will come to its original position. Hence hypertonic solutions may therefore be administered without permanent damage to the blood cells. They should be injected slowly to ensure rapid dilution into the blood stream and to minimise the crenulation of blood cells.

For the adjustment of tonicity of injectable solutions, substances like sodium chloride and dextrose etc. are added. About 0.9% solution of sodium chloride is isotonic, 0.45% solution is hypotonic and 5% solution of sodium chloride is hypertonic with plasma.

3.8 Calculations for Preparing Isotonic Solutions

For making isotonic solutions the quantities of substances to be added may be calculated by following methods :

1. Based on freezing point data.
2. Based on molecular concentration.
3. Graphical method based on vapour pressure and freezing point determinations.
4. Based on sodium chloride equivalents.

1. Based on Freezing Point Data

Freezing point is a physical property of solutions (also called coligative property) which is most often used in the calculations of isotonic solutions because it can be measured easily and accurately.

The temperature at which blood plasma and tears (lachrymal secretions) freeze is -0.52^{OC} which is the same value of a 0.9 per cent solution of sodium chloride. All solutions which freeze at -0.52^{OC} will be isotonic with blood plasma and lachrymal secretions. The freezing point of pure water is 0°C. The freezing point of a solution is also affected by the number of particles present in the solution. At the freezing point of water the liquid and the solid exist in equilibrium and have the same vapour pressure which ultimately lowers the freezing point of the liquid.

Adjustment to tonicity of solutions is simplified if the freezing point of medicament and the inert substance are known. The tables giving such informations are usually provided for reference. The freezing points are usually expressed in terms of 1% solutions. The quantity of adjusting substance needed for making the solutions isotonic with blood serum may be calculated from the general formula given below :

Percentage W/V of adjusting substance required

$$= \frac{0.52 - a}{b}$$

where a represents the freezing point of the unadjusted solution. *b* represents the freezing point of 1% W/V solution of the adjusting substance.

Each substance exerts its effect on the freezing point thus if two or more substances are present then the value of 'a' should be taken as sum of their depressions.

Table : The Freezing Point of a 1% W/V Solution of Substances Used in Solutions

Substance	*Freezing Point*	*Substance*	*Freezing point*
Adrenaline acid tartrate	–0.098 °C	Hyoscine hydrobromide	–0.068 °C
Apomorphine hydrocloride	–0.080 °C	Lignocaine hydrochloride	–0.130 °C
Atropine sulphate	–0.074 °C	Morphine hydrochloride	–0.086 °C
Benzalkonium chloride solution	–0.046 °C	Morphine sulphate	–0.079 °C
Boric acid	–0.288 °C	Neostigmine bromide	–0.127 °C
Calcium gluconate	–0.091 °C	Pethidine hydrochloride	–0.125 °C
Cocaine hydrochloride	–0.090 °C	Phenobarbitone sodium	–0.135 °C
Dextrose, anhydrous	–0.101 °C	Physostogmine salicylate	–0.090 °C
Dextrose, monohydrate	–0.091 °C	Pilocarpine nitrate	–0.132 °C
Emetine hydrochloride	–0.058 °C	Procaine hydrochloride	–0.122 °C
Homatropinehydrobromide	–0.097 °C	Silver nitrate	–0.190 °C
		Sodium chloride	–0.576 °C
		Sodium metabisulphite	–0.386 °C
		Sulphacetamide sodium	–0.132 °C

Example 1

Find the concentration of procaine hydrochloride required to make a solution isotonic with blood plasma. The freezing point of 1% W/V solution of procaine hydrochloride is -0.122°C.

By applying the general formula

$$\frac{0.52 - a}{b}$$

'a' the freezing point of unadjusted solution = 0.00°C

'b' the freezing point of 1% W/V solution of the adjusting substance

= – 0.122 °C

∴ Percentage W/V of procaine hydrochloride required

$$= \frac{0.52 - 0.00}{0.122} = 4.26\%\ \text{W/V}$$

Example 2

Find the concentration of sodium chloride required to render 1% solution of cocaine hydrochloride isotonic with blood plasma. The freezing point of 1% W/V solution of cocaine hydrochloride is -0.090°C and that of sodium chloride is -0.576°C.

By applying the general formula

$$\frac{0.52 - a}{b}$$

'a' the freezing point of unadjusted solution i.e. cocaine hydrochloride = -0.090°C

'b' the freezing point of 1% W/V solution of adjusted solution i.e. sodium chloride = -0.576°C

∴ Percentage W/V of sodium chloride required

$$\frac{0.52 - 0.090}{0.576} = 0.746\%\ \text{W/V}$$

Example 3

What concentration of sodium chloride will be required to make a 2% solution of procain hydrochloride isotonic with blood plasma. The freezing of 1% W/V solution of sodium chloride is –0.576 °C and that of procaine hydrochloride is -0.122°C.

By applying the general formula

$$\frac{0.52 - a}{b}$$

'a' the freezing point of 1% solution of unadjusted solution i.e. procaine hydrochloride is -0.012°C.

'b' the freezing point of 1% W/V solution of adjusted solution i.e. sodium chloride is -0.576°C

∴ Percentage W/V of sodium chloride required

$$= \frac{0.52 - (0.122 \times 2.0)}{0.576}$$

$$= \frac{0.52 - 0.244}{0.576} = 0.479\% \text{ W/V}$$

2. Based on Molecular Concentration

Freezing point of a solution depends on the concentration of the solute dissolved in it. Greater the concentration of the solute lower will be the freezing point. Thus the freezing point depends on the concentration of gram molecules of the solute, which ultimately depends on number of ions, molecular weight and weight of the substance.

If one gramme molecule of any non-ionising substance is dissolved in 100 gm of water the resulting solution will be of 1% gramme molecular concentration. For example the molecular weight of urea is 60, if 60 gm of urea are dissolved in 100 gm of water the resulting solution will have 1% molecular concentration.

An aqueous solution having 1% molecular concentration depresses the freezing point to -18.6°C and the freezing point of blood plasma is –0.52^{OC}. Therefore the molecular concentration of blood plasma and lachrymal secretions can be determined as follows :

A depression of 18.6°C is given by a mol. conc. of = 1%

A depression of 1°C is given by a mol. conc. of = $\frac{1}{18.6}$

∴ A depression of 0.52°C is given by a mol. conc. of

$$= \frac{1}{18.6} \times 0.52 = @\ 0.03\%$$

Hence any solution which have a molecular concentration of 0.03% will be isotonic with blood plasma and tears.

The formula for calculating the W/V per cent of non-ionising substance required to make the solution isotonic with blood plasma is as follows :

W/V percent of substance required = 0.03 × gramme molecular weight of the substance

The formula for calculating W/V per cent of ionising substance required to make the solution isotonic with blood plasma is therefore :

W/V per cent of substance required

$$= \frac{0.03 \times \text{gramme molecular weight of the substance}}{\text{number of ions yielded by the substance}}$$

Example 4

Calculate the quantity of dextrose required to make a solution isotonic with blood plasma. The mol. wt. of dextrose is 180 and is nonionising.

By applying the formula

W/V per cent of dextrose required

= 0.03 x gramme mol. wt. of dextrose

= 0.03 x 180

= 5.4%

Therefore 5.4 gm of dextrose is required for making 100 ml solution isotonic with blood plasma.

Example 5

Find the proportion of boric acid required to make a solution isotonic with tears. The mol. wt. of boric acid is 62 and is non-ionising.

By applying the formula.

W/V per cent of boric acid required

= 0.03 x gramme mol. wt. of boric acid

= 0.03 x 62

= 1.86%

Therefore 1.86 gm of boric acid is required to make 100 ml solution isotonic with tears (lachrymal secretions).

Example 6

Calculate the percentage of sodium chloride required to make a solution isotonic with blood plasma. The mol. wt. of sodium chloride is 58.5 and it yields 2 ions.

By applying the formula.

W/V per cent of sodium chloride required

$$= \frac{0.03 \times \text{ gm. mol. wt. of sodium chloride}}{\text{number of ions yielded by shodium chloride}}$$

$$= \frac{0.03 \times 58.5}{2}$$

$$= 0.88\% \ @ \ 0.90\%$$

Officially 0.9 gm of sodium chloride is used for making 100 ml solution isotonic with blood plasma.

3 Graphical Method

In this method a number of solutions of different concentrations of sodium chloride are prepared. The freezing points of all these solutions are determined very carefully and accurately. The solutions are used as standards. These standards are compared with solutions of common medicaments by using vapour pressure method.

From the data obtained, an accurate graph is prepared by plotting freezing point against concentration, for each medicament. Then on the same graph the curve for adjusting substance is also drawn, from where the percentage of adjusting substance required to make any percentage of medicament, isotonic with blood plasma can be determined.

4. Based on Sodium Chloride Equivalents

The sodium chloride equivalent method has gained popularity. Tables are used to find the concentration of sodium chloride needed to make a solution of a particular drug isotonic with blood plasma.

The value of sodium chloride equivalent is noted from the table provided, to the percentage of medicament in solution. This value is multiplied by the percentage of medicament. The result so obtained is subtracted from 0.9 per cent (the concentration of sodium chloride which will make the solution isotonic with blood plasma), the difference in values is the percentage of sodium chloride required to adjust the tonicity of the solutions.

Example 7

Find the proportion of sodium chloride required to make a 0.5% solution of potassium chloride isotonic with blood plasma. Sodium chloride equivalent of 0.5% potassium chloride is 0.76.

By applying the formula

Amount of sodium chloride required

= 0.9 - (0.5 x 0.76)

= 0.9 - 0.38

= 0.52%

Therefore 0.52 gm of sodium chloride is required to make 100 ml solution isotonic with blood plasma.

Answers.

(A)

1. 3 gr of Atropine sulphate to be dissolved in sufficient water to produce 330 m
2. Take 1 gr Acriflavine and dissolve it in sufficient water to produce 550 m. Out of this measure out 480 m and mix it with 480 m alcohol. Produce the final volume to 2 oz because there will be little contraction in volume which occurs when alcohol is diluted with water.
3. 1.750
4. 70.0 gr
5. 0.875 gr
6. 10.9375 gr
7. 157.5 gr
8. 4 tablets
9. 70 gr, 1120 gr
10. 17.5 gr, 280 gr

11. 109.375 gr, two tablespoonful to be diluted to a quart.

12. 262.5 gr, two teaspoonful to be diluted to 30 oz.

13. 1/8 oz or 60 minims

14. 1/4 oz or 120 minims

(B)

1. Dissolve 100 mg Potassium permanganate in sufficient water to produce 500 ml solution.
2. Dissolve 2 gm Acriflavine in sufficient water to produce 100 ml solution.
3. Dissolve 4.5 gm sodium chloride in sufficient water to produce 500 ml solution.
4. 150 ml
5. 231.578 ml
6. 126.315 ml
7. 105.263 ml
8. 266.666 ml
9. 1.5 lit
10. 113.636 gm.
11. 72.72 gm
12. 181.818 gm.

4

Packaging of Pharmaceuticals

Packaging is the process by which the pharmaceuticals are suitably packed so that they should retain their therapeutic effectiveness from the time of their packaging till they are consumed. Packaging may be defined as the art and science which involves preparing the articles for transport, storage, display and use. An utmost care might have been taken during the formulation of any preparation but if it is not packaged properly the whole aim may be lost. Different shapes and sizes of containers made from different materials are used for packing different types of formulations. Therefore a careful consideration must be given for the selection of packaging material. A package may consist of :

(i) Container. A container may be defined as a device in which the drug is enclosed and is in direct contact with the drug. A container which remains in contact with the drug at all times is known as immediate container.

(ii) Closure. A closure is a device which seals the container to exclude oxygen, carbon dioxide, moisture, micro-organisms and prevent the loss of volatile substances. It also prevents the loss of medicament during transport and handling. A closure is considered as a part of container system. It does not come in direct contact with the medicament.

(iii) Carton. Carton is the outer covering which gives secondary protection against mechanical and other environmental hazards. They are made from cardboard, moulded wood pulp or expanded polystyrene.

(iv) Box. A box is a device which is generally used for packing multiples of the product. It gives primary protection against external hazards during transport and handling. A box is usually made from thick cardboard, wood or any other suitable material.

4.1 Characteristics of Containers and Closures

1. The container must be sufficiently strong to withstand handling while empty, when filling, closing, sterilizing, labelling, transport, storage and use by the consumer.
2. They should not allow any loss of product due to leakage, spillage or permeation.
3. The material of the container from which they are prepared must not react with the contents.
4. They must be able to withstand heat if process includes sterilization by heat.
5. The surface of the container must be clear for easy labelling.
6. The container must not absorb substances from the preparation e.g. absorption of water and oily substances from ointments and creams by the cardboard boxes.
7. The container must not impart its own colour, taste and odour to the preparation.
8. The container and closure must not react either with each other or with the preparation.
9. The container should be able to protect light sensitive preparations for which amber coloured glass containers may be used.
10. The size of the container must be selected according to the size of the preparation.
11. The closure must be easy to remove and replace.
12. The cost of container and closure is an integral part of overall cost of the preparation, so it should not be high.
13. A container should facilitate the identification of a product i.e. whether meant for internal or external use.

14. Apart from all these characteristics a container and closure should be attractive in appearance and must have sale promotional and marketing values.

According to the method of closure and use, the containers are of following types :

1. Well Closed Containers

A well closed container is used to protect the preparation from contamination by extraneous solids, to prevent the loss of potency of active constituents and to prevent the loss of contents during transport, storage and handling.

2. Air-Tight Containers

Air-tight containers are used to protect the containers from atmospheric contamination of liquids, solids or vapours. They prevent the loss of drugs due to efflorescence, deliquescence or evaporation.

3. Hermetically-Sealed Containers

Hermetically-sealed container is that which does not allow the air and other gases to pass through it. Generally these types of containers are used for injectables. A glass ampoule sealed by fusion is the most common example of these types of containers.

4. Light Resistant Containers

Light resistant containers are used to protect the drugs which undergo decomposition in the presence of light. such drugs may be enclosed in light resistant amber coloured or opaque containers.

5. Single Dose Containers

They are used to supply only one dose of the medicament. They are sealed in such a way that the contents cannot be removed without removing the seal, the contents so removed are consumed immediately e.g. ampoules.

6. Multi Dose Containers

A multi dose container holds a number of doses. It is sealed in such a way that successive doses can be withdrawn easily without changing the strength, quality or purity of the remaining contents e.g. multidose vials.

7. Aerosol Containers

Containers for aerosols must be strong enough to withstand the pressure evolved inside the container at the time of use of the preparation.

4.2 Classification of Containers according to their shapes

1. Glass/polythene bottles
   (i) Narrow mouth
   (ii) Wide mouth
2. Dropper bottles
3. Collapsible tubes
4. Gallipots
5. Cardboard boxes
6. Ampoules
7. Vials
8. Polythene packets for intravenous fluids.
9. Polythene bottles for intravenous fluids.
10. Aerosol containers
11. Envelops, strips, cartons, boxes, drums etc.

Liquid oral preparations, intended to be swallowed like mixtures, emulsions, linctuses, syrups, oral gels, draughts etc. are required to be dispensed in narrow mouth bottles made from glass or polythene.

Liquid preparations, which are not to be swallowed like gargles, throat paints and mouth washes should be packed in fluted or ribbed bottles so that from its characteristic feel the patient may come to know that the preparation is not to be swallowed.

Liquid preparations like applications, liniments, lotions, paints etc. meant for external application to the skin should generally be supplied in coloured fluted bottles in order to distinguish them from preparations meant for internal use.

Eye drops, ear drops, nasal drops etc. should be dispensed in amber coloured glass bottles fitted with a dropper. Now a days manufacturers prefer a plastic squeeze bottle with a plastic cap to which a dropper device is attached. This type of arrangement has the advantage that whole of the medicament is not exposed to atmospheric conditions, when in use; the entire medicament is not contaminated as a few drops are instilled into the cavity while the dropper is still in its position; the chances of spillage of liquid from the container are eliminated.

Semisolid preparations like ointments, creams, pastes etc. are dispensed in wide mouth containers or gallipots. On manufacturing scale collapsible tubes made from metal or plastic are preferred because :

(i) Their narrow opening prevents the contamination of rest of the contents because the material once removed from the tube cannot re-enter it.

(ii) Wastage is reduced because patient will remove only the required amount of medicament.

(iii) Nozzle type applicators may be attached to the tube to facilitate introduction into the body cavities such as nose, vagina or anus.

Individual powders are dispensed in paperboard or plastic boxes or paperboard cartons. Bulk powders and granules for internal use are usually packed in wide mouth, screw capped, colourless glass jars but plastic containers and paper lined aluminium containers may also be used.

Dusting powders and insufflations are dispensed in air tight, wide mouthed, glass or plastic jars with instructions to the patient to use the powder with a swab of clean cotton wool or gauge. Proprietary dusting powders are packed in metal sifter-top containers.

Solid dosage forms like tablets, lozenges, hard and soft capsules are generally packed in strips made from cellophane or tin foil. For bulk packing either amber coloured vials or bottles are used which are closed with plastic or metal screw caps that contain a suitable insert. Suppositories and pessaries prepared by compression may be packed similar to that of tablets or capsules but suppositories prepared by moulding are wrapped individually in waxed paper or tin foil which is then packed in shallow partitioned paperboard boxes. Now a days suppositories are prepared in a strip of disposable plastic moulds.

4.3 Materials used for the construction of containers

The following materials are used for the construction of containers. They are used either singly or sometimes in combination with each other.

1. Glass
2. Plastics
3. Metals
4. Paper.

1. Glass

Glass is mostly produced by heating a mixture of silica (SiO_2), soda ash (Na_2CO_3) and lime stone ($CaCO_3$) in a furnace at about 1400°C. The fused mass on rapid cooling forms glass which is soft in nature and is used for making bottles, light bulbs etc. But if potassium carbonate is used instead of sodium carbonate, a hard glass is produced which is used for the preparation of laboratory glass apparatus. Special types of glass e.g. coloured glass or heat-resistant glass can be produced by adding certain other substances to the three basic components. Various types of glass used for pharmaceutical purposes are :

(a) Type I-Borosilicate glass
(b) Type II-Treated soda-lime glass
(c) Type III-Soda-lime glass
(d) Type NP-Non-parenteral glass
(e) Coloured glass
(f) Neutral glass

(a) Type I — Borosilicate Glass

Borosilicate glass is produced by replacing the sodium oxide flux by boric oxide (B_2O_3) and some of lime by alumina (Al_2O_3) in the basic components of glass. It has a high melting point and can withstand high temperatures hence it does not crack when used for boiling the water and even for cooking.

It is also resistant to chemical substances. This type of glass is mainly used for making laboratory glass apparatus, in factories, kitchens and ovens.

(b) Type II — Treated Soda-lime Glass

It is prepared from commercial soda-lime glass by treating it with sulphur dioxide by which surface alkali is de-alkanised and such glass can be used for alkali sensitive products.

Sometimes inner surface of glass is treated with silicones and the glass so treated can be used for alkali sensitive products. Silicon treated glass is not very popular with pharmaceutical manufacturers due to flaking.

(c) Type III — Soda Lime Glass

It is an ordinary glass prepared from silicon dioxide, soda ash (for Na_2O) and lime stone (for CaO) and is generally referred to as soda lime glass. It is the cheapest quality and most common form of glass. It contains a high concentration of alkaline oxides and imparts alkalinity to aqueous substances readily which can adversely effect the quality of the product contained therein. So these types of glasses are not suitable for alkali sensitive products. They should not be used for parenteral preparations. These types of containers are generally used for solid medicaments.

(d) Type NP — Non-parenteral Glass

It is general purpose soda-lime glass used for oral and topical preparations.

(e) Coloured Glass

Coloured glass is obtained by adding small amounts of metal salts during fusion of glass. Coloured glass is used for light sensitive products. For this purpose amber coloured glass is generally used which does not allow the U.V. rays to pass through it. Preferably coloured glass should not be used for parenteral products because it becomes difficult to check clarity in such preparations.

(f) Neutral Glass

It is another commercial variety of glass available in between sodalime glass and borosilicate glass. It is resistant to alkalies, weathering; and can withstand autoclaving. It is used for the manufacture of multidose vials and transfusion bottles etc. It is composed of SIO_2 75%, B_2O_3 7-10%, Na_2O 6-8%, Al_2O_3 4-6%, BaO 2-4%, K_2O 0.5-2%.

For the manufacture of ampoules special glass tubing having low melting point should be used because after filling the ampoules are required to be sealed by fusion of glass.

Flaking

During flaking the alkali is extracted from the surface of glass containers and a silica rich layer is formed which sometimes gets detached from the surface and can be seen in the contents in the form of shining flakes. This is a serious problem specially in parenteral preparations. Therefore glass which does not flake should be selected.

Weathering

Weathering is a common problem with glass containers, that sometimes moisture condensed on the surface of glass container, can extract some weakly bounded alkali, leaving behind a white deposit of alkali carbonate. If this white deposit is not removed and allowed to remain over there, further condensation of moisture will lead to the formation of an alkaline solution which will dissolve some silica resulting in loss of brilliance. This loss of brilliance from the surface of glass is called weathering. To prevent weathering, the deposited white layer of alkali carbonates should be removed as early as possible by washing the container with a dilute solution of acid and then washing thoroughly with water.

Sometimes glass free from lead and arsenic is used for those preparations which can extract lead or arsenic from the containers.

Due to flaking and weathering, all the glass apparatuses used for pharmaceutical purposes must be free from alkali and all the containers used therein must have passed the limit tests for alkalinity as prescribed in various pharmacopoeias.

Advantages of Glass Containers

1. They are transparent which allows the visual inspection of the contents.
2. They are economical.
3. They are readily available in various shapes and sizes.
4. They are chemically inert.
5. They are quite strong and rigid.
6. They possess superior protection properties.
7. They do not deteriorate with age, with proper closures.
8. Some glass containers are heat resistant so they can be readily sterilized by heat.
9. Glass containers can be easily cleaned without any damage to its surface e.g. scratching or bruising.
10. As the composition of glass may be varied by adding suitable amounts and types of sand and silica as well as conditions of heat treatment used, the proper container according to desired qualities can be produced.

Disadvantages

1. They are brittle and break easily.
2. They may crack when subjected to sudden changes of temperatures.
3. Some containers impart alkalinity and insoluble flakes to the formulations. This type of difficulty can be overcome by selecting proper type of glass.

2. Plastics

Plastics are high molecular weight polymers possessing long carbon chains. They are synthetic polymers which are converted into different forms. There are two types of plastics (i) thermosetting type (ii) thermoplastic type.

The thermosetting type plastics are usually hard and brittle at room temperature but become flexible on heating. They are used for making the closures for bottles and jars.

The thermoplastic type plastics are becoming more popular day be day. This type of plastic is used for the manufacture of plastic containers which are mainly used for packing mixtures, tablets, capsules, ointments etc. I/V fluids and retention enemas are now packaged in plasticised PVC 'sachet' packs. These types of plastics have characteristic property that on heating they soften to become viscous fluids while on cooling again hardens. The various thermoplastic polymers used for the manufacture of containers are :

(i) Low density polythene It is used for the manufacture of bottles, jars, collapsible tubes etc.

(ii) High density polythene It is also used for bottles, jars and closures.

(iii) Polyvinyl chloride (PVC) It is of two types :

(a) Unplasticised which is used for bottles and jars.

(b) Plasticised which is used for making extruded tubes and films.

(iv) Polystyrene It is used for jars tubes and closures etc. but is not suitable for the moisture sensitive products.

(v) Polypropylene It is used for the manufacture of squeeze bottles. It has a melting point of 170°C and containers made from it can be sterilized by autoclaving. It has a drawback that it becomes brittle at low temperatures.

(vi) Polymethylmethacrylate (PMMA) It is clear, hard, strong and light and is used for the manufacture of bottles, tubes etc. It has the drawback that at low temperatures it becomes soft therefore not very suitable for containers of sterile products.

(vii) Polytetrafluoroethylene (PTFE) It has high resistance to heat and can withstand a temperature upto 250°C. It is also resistant to chemicals and its permeability to water vapours is also very low. It is very costly due to which it is not so commonly used in pharmaceutical practice.

(viii) Polyamides (Nylons) Nylons are very tough materials but at the same time they are also very flexible. They are resistant to heat with melting point of about 200 °C. They are also resistant to chemicals. Nylons can be easily sterilized by autoclaving.

Sometimes in addition to above mentioned basic polymers, other additives such as plasticizers, anti-oxidants, colouring agents etc. may be incorporated. Since these additives do not form bonds with the basic polymers so they may transmit to the preparation on storage, resulting to spoil the product.

Before packing the pharmaceutical products into the plastic containers they must be physically, chemically and biologically tested to ensure safety and stability of the preparation. The containers must be free from toxicity, irritability and pyrogens etc., whenever necessary. Plastic containers meant for photosensitive materials, should be tested for penetration of ultra-violet rays. Whenever coloured containers are used, it must be ensured that the colour is not transmitted to the preparation.

Advantages of Plastic Containers

1. They are cheaper as compared to other containers.
2. They can be readily produced on large scale.
3. They are unbreakable, tough and flexible.
4. They are light in weight and can be easily transported.
5. They can be moulded into various shapes and sizes.

3. Metals

Metal containers are not very popular for packing the pharmaceutical products because they may react with the preparations, have considerable weight and are costlier. Metal containers are however, used for packing aerosols, powders, tablets and food articles. For this purpose tin plated steel, stainless steel and aluminium containers are used.

Collapsible tubes made from aluminium, tin and lead are used but aluminium tubes are most popular because they are cheap as compared to tubes made from tin. Collapsible tubes are used for packing ointments, creams, pastes, tooth pastes and cosmetics. They are attractive containers and allow only the desired amount of the product to be removed. They do not allow the product to be contaminated as the rest of the preparation will not come in contact neither with the fingers nor with the atmosphere. Collapsible tubes are light in weight, unbreakable and can be filled easily at a high speed with automatic machines.

Collapsible tubes are available in different sizes. Sometimes they are supplied with nozzles which can be attached to the tube for ease in application of the medicament to the nose, rectum or other body cavities.

4. Paper

Paper and board as packing material are widely used in pharmaceutical industries in one form or the other. They are used to prepare containers ranging from envelops used for dispensing powders, a few tablets or a few capsules on the counter, to the drums used for storing large quantities of drugs in the industries. Cartons and boxes made from board are used for packing the pharmaceutical containers.

Properties of paper and board can be modified by treating it with plastic, wax or other materials. Such treated paper will protect the products from atmospheric conditions. Now a days chemically treated paper known as tetra pack paper is also available for storing the drugs and chemicals.

Materials Used for the Construction of Closures

1. Cork
2. Glass
3. Plastics
4. Rubber
5. Metals

1. Cork

Cork is essentially a wood obtained from the bark of oak tree. It is used for the manufacture of stoppers for narrow mouth bottles. Cork is almost chemically inert and do not impart undesirable odour or flavour to the preparation. The main disadvantage of these closures is that sometimes they lead to mould growth when used for aqueous preparations and may shed particles to products if not used carefully.

2. *Glass*

As compared to cork, glass is an ideal material for making the stoppers but these stoppers have the difficulties that they do not provide leak proof closures moreover they can slip out of neck of the containers easily during transport and handling. Therefore the use of glass closures is restricted to laboratory glass apparatus e.g. reagent bottles and fancy cut glass items only.

3. *Plastics*

As compared to cork, glass, rubber and metal closures, plastic closures are becoming more popular day by day because they are unbreakable, light in weight, can be easily moulded into various shapes and sizes. Plastic closures selected must be tested before use for any extractive material present in them and for their reaction with the product contained in the bottle.

4. *Rubber*

Natural rubber consists of latex obtained from Heavea braziliensis commonly known as rubber plant. This rubber imparts a characteristic odour to the product therefore the physical and chemical properties of rubber are altered by the addition of some additives such as :

(a) Vulcanising agent e.g. sulphur.

(b) Accelerators e.g. thiazoles.

(c) Activators e.g. zinc oxide, stearic acid and zinc stearate.

(d) Fillers e.g. carbon black, calcium carbonate, zinc oxide, talc etc.

(e) Softners e.g. mineral oils etc.

(f) Antioxidants.

(g) Pigments e.g. oxides and sulphides of iron, cadmium etc.

(h) Lubricants e.g. zinc stearate etc.

Rubber closures are mainly used for vials, multidose containers and I/V fluid bottles because of its self sealing properties and it can withstand sterilization temperatures better than plastic closures. Rubber is also used for making the washers required in certain containers.

Since the additives used in the manufacture of rubber has the tendency to migrate into the product contained in the container therefore these closures must be subjected to extractive test before use. The other tests which should be performed on rubber closures include (i) test for penetrability force (ii) fragmentation test (iii) permeability test and compatibility with the product.

Qualities of an Ideal Rubber Closure

(i) It should provide air tight closing to the container.
(ii) It should be compatible with the preparation contained in the container.
(iii) It should not migrate any additive to the preparation.
(iv) It should withstand the sterilization temperatures.
(v) It should be soft and elastic in nature so as to allow the hypodermic needle to pass through it easily but as soon as the needle is removed it should again provide the perfect seal.

Synthetic rubbers are costly so not very commonly used for the manufacture of closures.

Advantages of rubber

1. Rubber does not deteriorate with age. Under normal conditions closures prepared from good quality rubber remain stable for a number of years.
2. Rubber acts as self seal to the containers.
3. Rubber is elastic in nature and can be moulded in any form to make stoppers or closure liners. It is elastic enough that it provides a snug fit between the closure and the neck and lip of the glass container. They are soft and elastic enough that they allow easy passage to the syringe needle without blunting and springs back to its original position to close the hole made by the needle immediately after withdrawal to prevent the entry of micro-organisms and leakage of the contents.

4. Although porous they do not allow the transfer of water vapours or gases in either direction.
5. Good quality rubber is resistant to sterilization conditions.
6. They are unbreakable, tough and can be easily transported.

Disadvantages of rubber :

1. The composition of rubber stoppers is complex and the manufacture process is complicate.
2. When rubber stopper comes in contact with parenteral solutions, it may absorb the active medicament, preservative or other materials, and one or more constituents of the rubber may be extracted into the liquid which may (a) interfere with the chemical analysis of the active medicament, (b) affect the toxicity or pyrogenicity of the parenteral preparation, (c) lose or decrease the preservation and physical stability of the preparation
3. Hard rubber may produce large number of fragments when the hypodermic needle cuts through the closure and the fragmented material may appear in the solution.

5. Metals

Tin plate and aluminium are most commonly used for the manufacture of closures but aluminium is most widely used for this purpose because it is ductile in nature and closure of any desired shape and size can be easily manufactured with it. Further, tear off closures can only be made from aluminium. To make the closures pilfer-proof they may be sealed with aluminium cap in such a way that its central part is easily removed at the time of administration of the preparation but the cap itself should remain in position, if so desired.

4.4 Closure Liners

Closure liners are the materials which are placed in a closure to make it pilfer-proof and prevent the decomposition of the product due to moisture, bacterial or fungal growth.

Almost all types of closures except glass stoppers must be packed with a suitable liner which may include cork, rubber, pulp board, plastic and felt.

Types of closures

1. Once-only closures e.g. fusion of glass to seal an ampoule or fusion of plastic to seal a polyethylene bag.
2. Renewable cloures-they are used for bottles, jars, tubes etc. and is of following types :
   (a) *Plug type* e.g. closing the neck of the container with a cork or glass stopper but both of these have been replaced by plastic stoppers because they are unbreakable and flexible to ensure better fitting.
   (b) *Cap type*
   (i) *Push fit caps* e.g. closing of the tablet or capsule vials where the neck of the container and plastic cap is shaped in such a way that the cap fit well in the neck of the container and cap is stretched over it so as to provide a perfect seal.
   (ii) *Screw closures* - they are the most widely used closures for all types of containers having screwed neck but care must be taken that the cap should also be screwed to the correct extent.

4.5 Strip or Blister Packaging

Unit dosage form of drugs like tablets and capsules are enclosed individually in strip or blister packs. In strip packing the unit drugs are hermetically sealed in between strips of aluminium foil and/or plastic film. the contents are removed by tearing or cutting the individual pocket.

In blister packing the unit dosage forms are enclosed in between transparent blisters and suitable backing material, generally aluminium foil. The contents are removed simply by pushing the drug through the backing strip.

4.6 Aerosols

A pharmaceutical aerosol may be defined as the preparation containing the active medicament dissolved, suspended or emulsified in a propellant or a mixture of solvent and propellant and packaged in a pressurised aerosol container. When little pressure is applied on the valve attached to the pressurised container, the medicament is released in the form of a mist or an aerosol spray. For aerosol systems the propellants used include compressed gases such as carbon dioxide or nitrogen or liquefied gases like methane, ethane etc. Liquefied gases are more commonly used as propellants because they maintain a constant pressure until last drop of the product is taken out of the container. For potent drugs used in asthma the valve includes a metering device which delivers only a metered dose on applying pressure on the valve. The patients should be warned not to exceed the prescribed dose.

Uses

Pressurised aerosols are becoming more popular day by day. They are used only in pharmaceutical practice but a large number of consumer items like cosmetics, perfumes etc. are being packed in pressure aerosol containers inspite of high packing costs. Pharmaceutical pressurised aerosols are used as local applications, local anaesthetics, local analgesics, antiseptics, germicides, antibiotics, anti-inflammatory agents, local application to the ear, nose, throat, lungs, etc.

Advantages of Aerosols

1. The products are easy and convenient to apply and can be administered without the help of a nurse or a doctor as is required in the case of injections.
2. The onset of action is faster because the medicament is directly administered to the affected part.
3. The dispersion of medicament is very efficient.
4. There is no manual contact with the medicament and the affected parts.

5. The possibility of drug decomposition in G.I.T. on oral administration is eliminated since no drug is to pass through G.I.T.
6. There is no contamination of the product from external sources.
7. The sterility of the sterile products is maintained since no micro-organism can enter even when the value is opened.
8. Controlled and uniform dose is released by the metered valves.
9. Hydrolysis of medicament can be prevented since propellants do not contain any water.
10. Oxidation is prevented as no air is present in the container.
11. The aerosol containers except clear glass containers protect the photosensitive medicaments.
12. A fine mist of the drug is produced for inhalation purposes.

Disadvantages of Aerosols

1. They are costlier.
2. The disposal of empty containers may be difficult because the remaining amount of propellant present in the exhausted containers continue to exert pressure.
3. Aerosol packs must not be exposed to higher temperatures because it may develop high pressure inside the container.
4. When the drug is not soluble in the propellant it may create difficulties in the formulation of aerosols.
5. Propellants may cause toxic reactions if inhalation therapy is continued for a long period of time.

Formulation of Pharmaceutical Aerosols

A pharmaceutical aerosol consists of following essential components :

(i) Active medicament
(ii) Solvent
(iii) Propellant

The active medicament(s) is dissolved in a suitable solvent to which other ingredients such as stabilizers, antioxidants, preservatives, solubilizers or dispersing agents may be incorporated. To this a propellant or a blend of propellants is added to develop pressure inside the container and to expel the product from the container when the valve is opened. Propellants can be mixed with active medicaments in a number of ways, producing products with different characteristics. Various gases used as aerosol propellants include :

(i) Compressed gases like carbon dioxide, nitrogen and nitrous oxide. Out of these only nitrogen is more useful in aerosols because it is inert.

(ii) Liquefied gases include fluorinated and fluorochlorinated hydrocarbons. Although a large number of compounds are available but dichlorodifluoromethane, trichloromonofluoromethane and dichlorotetrafluoroethane are widely used propellants in most pharmaceutical aerosols.

Aerosol Containers

An aerosol container assembly consists of following parts:

(i) Container

(ii) Valve

(i) *Container* The container used for packaging the pharmaceutical aerosols must possess at least the following qualities that (a) it should be capable of maintaining the required high pressure (b) the material from which it is manufactured must be compatible with the contents. The aerosol containers are generally made from tin plate, aluminium, glass, plastic coated glass and plastics. In addition to all these materials, stainless steel is used in special cases to prevent attack by the contents.

(ii) *Valve* The valve mechanism is the most important part of an aerosol assembly. Its main function is to regulate the flow of the product from the container and to control the type of spray. The valve includes not only the basic valve mechanism but it includes the closure in which it is mounted, the gasket, the dip tube and the actuator.

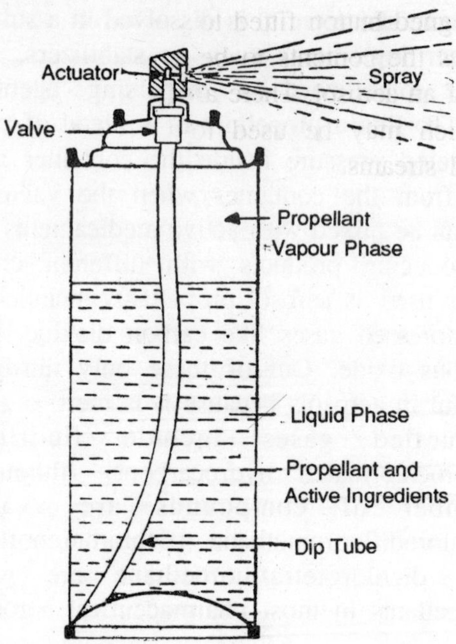

Fig. 4.1 Aerosol container

Various types of valves are used in aerosols which include (a) continuous spray valves and (b) metering valves. In continuous spray valves the medicament is continuously released from the container unless the pressure is released from the actuator. Such valves include spray valves used for spray aerosols e.g. room deodorants, anaesthetics, disinfectants etc; foam valves used for foam producing aerosols e.g. shaving creams, vaginal contraceptive foam aerosols etc.; stream valves used for solid stream aerosols, e.g. tooth pastes, ointments, creams etc.

Metered valves are used for potent drugs where a measured quantity of drug is required to be administered during each single operation of the actuator. These type of valves minimize the wastage and errors of overdosing of drugs.

An actuator is an integral part of each aerosol container which allows easy opening and closing of the valve. It is a specially designed button fitted to the valve stem which when pressed allows the contents to be released from the container in the form of an aerosol. There are different types of actuators available which may be used to produce spray, fine mist, foam or solid streams.

5
Size Reduction

Size reduction is the process of reducing the particle size of a substance to a finer state of subdivision to smaller pieces, to coarse particles or to powder. Comminution and grinding are the synonym terms used for the process of size reduction. When the particle size of solids is reduced by mechanical means it is known as milling.

Very rarely, the materials to be used in pharmaceutical formulations exist in the optimum size therefore majority of them will have to be reduced to a desired size at one stage or the other during the formulation of a dosage form. There are a large number of processes which are used in size reduction e.g. cutting, chopping, crushing, grinding, milling, micronizing and trituration which depends on the type of equipment employed. The selection of an equipment depends on the properties of the material to be reduced, initial particle size and degree of size reduction required.

5.1 Pharmaceutical Applications of Size Reduction

1. Size reduction increases the surface area of drugs which helps in rapid solution formation in the case of chemical substances.
2. With increase in surface area the extraction from animal glands such as liver and pancreas and from crude vegetable drugs is facilitated because solvent can easily penetrate into the tissues resulting in quick extraction of their active constituents.

3. The therapeutic effectiveness of certain drugs is increased by reducing the particle size e.g. the dose of griseofulvin is reduced to half than that of originally required.
4. The mixing of several solid ingredients is easier and more uniform if the ingredients are reduced to same particle size.
5. In the case of powdered pharmaceutical dosage forms it is important to powder the crystalline drugs before mixing them with other drugs in order to mix all the drugs uniformly and to avoid recognition of crystalline drugs by the patients.
6. In the manufacture of tablets relatively few drugs can be compressed directly, generally they are mixed with excipients and made in the form of suitable size granules which are then compressed.
7. The stability of emulsions is increased by decreasing the size of the oil globules.
8. In the case of suspensions the size of the particles play a great role. If the size of the particles is too small, they may form a cake which may not re-disperse easily but on the other hand large size particles settle quickly but form a loose cake which may re-disperse easily on shaking.
9. Appropriate particle size is used in the inhalations. Very small particles may be exhaled out of the bronchioles along with air without producing its effect.
10. The physical appearance of ointments, pastes and creams can be improved by reducing its particle size.
11. All the ophthalmic preparations and preparations meant for external application to the skin must be free from gritty particles to avoid irritation of the area to which they are applied.
12. The rate of absorption of a drug depends on the dosage form, route of administration and particle size. The smaller the particle size, quicker and greater will be rate of absorption.
13. Depending on the particle size, the sustained action of a preparation can be produced.

14. In certain drugs the colour and texture is changed on reducing the particle size.
15. The rate of drying is enhanced if the particle size is reduced.
16. On reducing the particle size the bulkiness of certain drugs can be increased.

5.2 Disadvantages

1. On grinding, the aromatic and volatile constituents of crude drugs may be lost due to increase in temperature during grinding. Therefore drugs such as cinnamon, clove, cardamom, caraway and other drugs containing volatile oils must not be subjected to heavy grinding to prevent the loss of volatile oils.
2. Since on size reduction the surface area is increased which when exposed to atmospheric conditions may result in oxidation and hydrolysis. Therefore such drugs must be stored in a well closed container and at a cool place.

5.3 Factors Affecting Size Reduction

The following factors should be taken into consideration while reducing the particle size of a drug :

1. Physical properties of drugs such as hardness, toughness, moisture content etc.
2. Melting or softening point of the material : The heat generated during mechanical grinding present many problems with materials which tend to liquefy, stick with each other; and with thermolabile substances.
3. The size of the starting material : If the size of the original drugs is too large it may be reduced to small particles in stages.
4. The quantity of the material to be reduced.
5. Size, shape, flow properties and bulk density of the reduced particles.
6. The solubility of the drug.
7. If the material is to be kept free from bacterial contamination, then the reduction will have to be carried out under aseptic conditions.

8. Overall costs of process involved including power consumption, space occupied, labour expenditure and time involved.

5.4 Methods of Size Reduction

The processes such as slicing and cutting, bruising and contusion, rasping or grating, chopping and grinding are less important today than were in the past. Now a days manufacturers use very well developed machines by which powders of desired degree of fineness can be obtained.

Certain vegetable drugs like stems, roots, barks, fruits and seeds may require preliminary size reduction therefore following methods may still be used :

1. Slicing and Cutting

Slicing and cutting may be done with a sharp knife, a pair of scissors, a root cutter or any other sharp instrument. It may be done either in transverse or longitudinal direction. This method is usually employed to hasten the drying of crude vegetable drugs such as leaves and roots. For cutting the drugs on a large scale a cutter mill is used.

Cutter Mill

Cutter mill is fitted with two types of knives i.e. stationary and rotating. The stationary knives are mounted in the casing of the machine and rotating knives are attached to a rotor which rotates at a high speed. The upper part is attached with a hopper and at the lower part of the machine a screen of desired size is attached.

The material to be reduced in size is put in the hopper and reduced material is collected from the screen. This method is used to obtain a coarse degree of size reduction of soft materials such as roots and peels before its extraction.

2. Bruising or Contusion

It is a process in which the particle size of the drugs is reduced by striking heavy blows in succession over the drug.

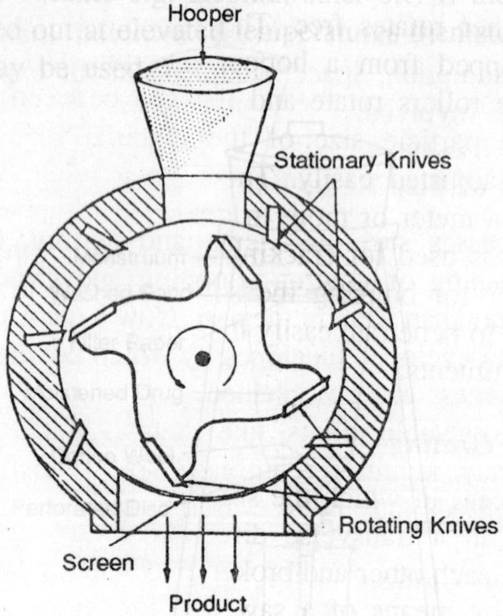

Fig. 5.1 Cutter mill

For this purpose ordinary porcelain pestle and mortar or steel pestle and mortar may be used. Porcelain pestle and mortar should not be used for drugs containing acidic constituents and steel pestle and mortar should not be used for drugs containing tannins. On large scale roller mill is used.

Roller Mill

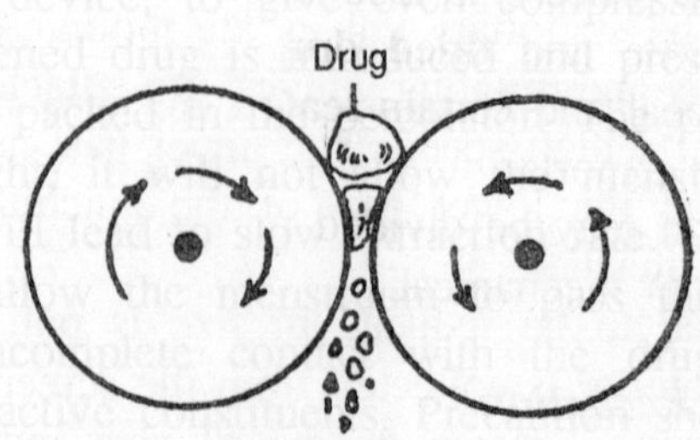

Fig. 5.2 Roller mill

Roller mill consists of two equal size rolls made up of stone or metal with an adjustable gap between them to control the size of the product. Generally one roll is driven mechanically whereas the other rotates free. The material to be bruised or crushed is dropped from a hopper into the gap. The speed with which the rollers rotate and the gap between the rollers determines the particle size of the material to be crushed, which can be adjusted easily. The rolls varying from a few centimeters to a meter or more in diameter are available.

Roller mill is used for cracking the seeds before extraction of fixed oils or for bruising the soft tissues in order to help the menstruum to penetrate easily thus facilitating the extraction of active constituents.

3. Rasping or Grating

It is a process in which the soft woody drugs or materials are thinly cut in a transverse direction which can be easily separated from each other and broken into small pieces. Rasping may be done by means of a saw and for large scale work a saw mill may be used. This process is used for a few drugs such as cocoa butter, quassia wood and certain waxes and soaps.

4. Grinding

It is a process in which the substances are reduced into coarse particles or fine powders. On small scale crystalline substances are usually reduced to a fine powder in a pestle and mortar. This process is also known as trituration. Small quantities of brittle and dried drugs such as aloe, catechu, coriander, cochineal and certain leaves etc. may be reduced to a fine powder in a mortar.

Size reduction may be divided into two general categories (i) manual and (ii) mechanical.

1. Manual Size Reduction

On small scale the size reduction may be carried out manually by means of :

(a) Trituration
(b) Levigation
(c) Pulverization by intervention.

(a) Trituration By trituration the grinding of a solid substance is done to a fine powder by continuous striking or rubbing the particles in a mortar with a pestle. The term trituration is also employed to designate the process by which two or more powders are intimately mixed with each other. For this purpose a pestle and mortar made of wedgewood ware, porcelain or glass is used. For hard materials steel pestle and mortar may be used.

(b) Levigation The process of levigation is also known as wet grinding. In this process the particle size of a substance is reduced to finer state of subdivision by triturating the substance with a few drops of a liquid in which it is insoluble, in a glass mortar with a pestle or on a slab with spatula or muller. The most commonly used levigating agents include oils, water, alcohol and glycerin.

This process is often used to incorporate solid substances into dermatological and ophthalmic ointments and suspensions. When a levigating agent is mixed with the solid ingredients of the ointment a paste is formed which should be further triturated until smooth product is obtained.

(c) Pulverization by intervention This is a process by which the solid substances are reduced to a fine powder by means of triturating the solid with a suitable solvent which can be easily removed at the end of the process. For example camphor is difficult to powder in a mortar because the particles tend to cohere as quickly as they are powdered. But when the camphor is triturated with a few drops of alcohol, ether or chloroform it can be powdered easily. The solvent added evaporates quickly leaving behind the finely subdivided particles of camphor. Similarly iodine crystals may be powdered with the help of a small quantity of ether.

2. Mechanical Size Reduction

For. large scale work, size reduction is carried out mostly by using different kind of mills which have the capability of producing powders with wide range of particle size. Since different mills are used for mechanical size reduction hence this process is also known as milling. Various mills used for this purpose are :

1. Ball mill
2. Hammer mill
3. Edge runner mill
4. End runner mill
5. The disintegrator
6. Bohr stone mill
7. Hand mill
8. Colloid mill
9. Fluid energy mill

5.5 Mechanisms of Size Reduction

(i) Cutting During this process the material is cut into small pieces by means of a sharp blade or any other sharp instrument.

(ii) Compression During this process the material is crushed by application of pressure with a suitable device.

(iii) Impact During impact the material which is more or less stationary, is hit by an object moving at a high speed or the moving particles strike a stationary surface and the material is broken into smaller particles.

(iv) Attrition During attrition the pressure is applied to the material as in the case of compression but the surfaces are in motion in relation to each other, resulting in shear forces which break the particles into still smaller particles.

1. Ball Mill

This mill works on the principle of impact and attrition.

The ball mill which is also called jar mill consists of a cylindrical container or jar made up of steel or porcelain. The length of the cylinder is slightly greater than its diameter which is partially filled with balls made from the same material as that of cylindrical vessel. The balls act as grinding medium. If pebbles, rods or bars are used in place of balls then the mill is known as pebble mill, rod mill or bar mill respectively. In a ball mill, generally the balls made from steel are used which are often the most efficient but may produce deterioration or contamination of certain substances therefore balls made of porcelain, flint, nylon or rubber may be used and the inner surface of cylindrical vessel is also lined with same type of material as that of balls.

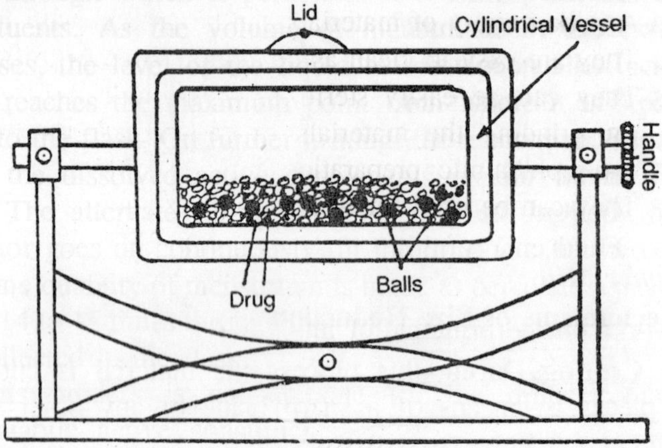

Fig. 5.3 Ball mill

The cylindrical vessel is mounted on a metallic frame and rotates horizontally by hand or mechanically. The upper side of the vessel is fitted with a tightly closed lid through which the material is introduced.

The material to be ground is put into the mill through the lid. The mill is rotated at a slow speed until the product of desired size is produced. Rotation of the mill at high speed is avoided because at high speed the balls are held against the mill casing by centrifugal force and revolve with the mill and will not fall on the drug when they reach at the top position. After an appropriate time when the material has been reduced it is taken out from the vessel and passed through a suitable sieve to get the powder of desired particle size. The particle size of the material is reduced by rolling, sliding and tumbling of the balls on the material to be reduced. The balls used are 2-5 cm in diameter. The smaller size balls are more efficient because they produce fine particles. The speed at which the ball mill is rotated is also important.

Ball mills are available in many sizes and designs and are also available for batch or continuous production.

Advantages

1. They are economical and simple to operate.

2. They afford a large grinding surface within a compact space.
3. A wide variety of materials can be ground with it.
4. They are easy to clean as compared to other mills.
5. They can be easily sterilized therefore can be used for grinding the materials to be used in parenteral and ophthalmic preparations.
6. They can be used for wet and dry grinding.

2. Hammer Mill

It works on the principle of impact.

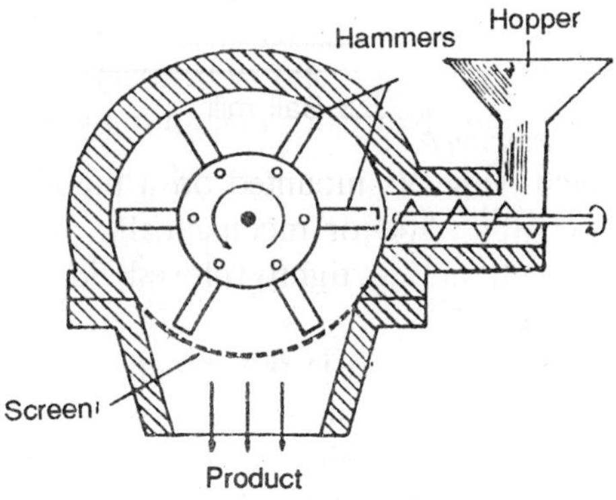

Fig. 5.4 Hammer mill

The hammer mill consists of a steel casing in which a central shaft is enclosed to which a number of swinging hammers are attached. When the shaft is rotated the hammers swing out to a radial position. On the lower part of the casing a screen of desired size is fitted which can be easily replaced according to the particle size required. The construction of a hammer mill is almost similar to that of a disintegrator with the difference that in hammer mill the hammers are swinging in nature which are mounted with swivel joints and in disintegrator the beaters or hammers are fixed. These mills are provided with a fan and a cyclone for collecting the material when it has been reduced to the desired size.

The material to be reduced in size is fed through the hopper which is then supplied to the mill centrifugally and reduced in size by impact of hammers or against the plates along the periphery of the mill casing. The reduced powder passes out through the screen fitted at the lower part of the mill and unreduced particles are retained in the mill for further reduction in size.

The hammer mills are available in various designs and shapes. In pharmaceutical industry they are used for grinding dry materials, wet filter cakes, ointments and slurries.

Advantages

1. They are simple to instal and operate, the operation is continuous.
2. They are rapid in action and many different types of materials can be ground with them.
3. There are no chances of contamination due to abration of metal from the mill because no surface of the mill move against each other.
4. The particle size of the material to be reduced can be easily controlled by changing the speed of the rotor, hammer type, shape and size of the screen.

3. Edge Runner Mill

This mill works on the principle of crushing and friction.

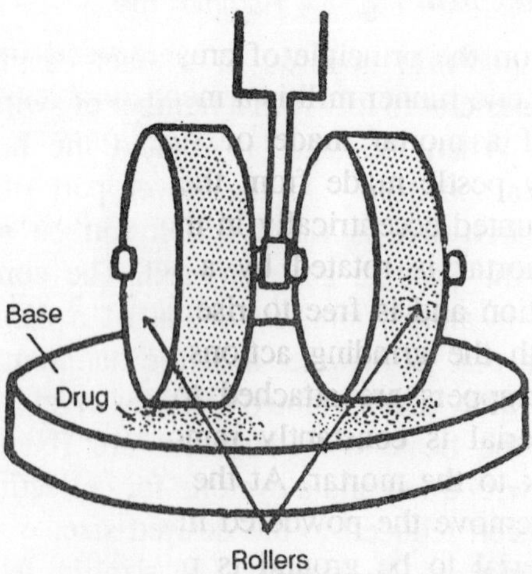

Fig. 5.5 Edge runner mill

The edge runner mill is also known as chaser mill because two heavy wheels made of steel or granite are mounted vertically on a horizontal shaft which are made to revolve or chase each other on a steel or granite base. The stones may vary from 0.5 to 2.5 meter in diameter. The large size rollers may weigh upto 6 tonnes, usually the wheels are rotated but sometimes the bed is made to rotate. The height between the rollers and the base determines the particle size of the material hence the fineness of the particles can be increased or decreased by adjusting the height.

The material to be ground is put on the base of the mill and is kept in the path of the runners by scrappers. The particle size is reduced due to crushing by the weight of rollers but is more due to the friction between the rollers and the bed stone. After grinding the material for a specified time it is taken out of the mill, passed through a suitable sieve and the coarse material obtained after sieving is again put in the mill for regrinding or it may be mixed with the material to be ground in the next batch.

Although the edge runner mills are being replaced with more sophisticated machines but still they are used to reduce the particle size of extremely tough and fibrous roots and barks.

4. End Runner Mill

It works on the principle of crushing and shearing.

Basically end runner mill is a mechanical pestle and mortar. It consists of a mortar made of steel or granite. A dumble shaped heavy pestle made from the same material as that of mortar is mounted eccentrically in the mortar through a hinged joint. The mortar is rotated by a motor. The pestle rotates itself by friction and is free to rise and fall in the mortar due to which both the grinding actions i.e. impact and shear are produced. Scrappers are attached to the pestle which ensure that the material is constantly removed from the pestle and returned back to the mortar. At the end of grinding the pestle is raised to remove the powdered material.

The material to be ground is put in the mortar which is rotated mechanically. The pestle rotates itself by friction. The material is crushed and rubbed between the pestle and rotating mortar. The scrappers remove the sticking material from the pestle and returns back to the mortar for grinding. At the end of grinding the pestle is raised to facilitate emptying and cleaning of the mortar. The ground material is passed through a sieve to get the powder of required particle size.

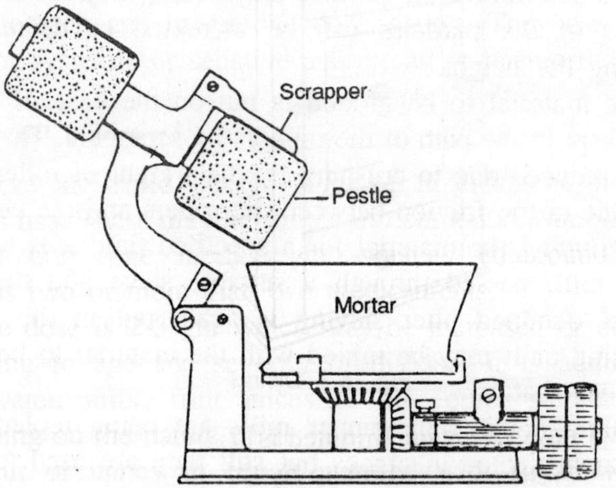

Fig. 5.6 End runner mill

Advantages

This mill is quite suitable for reducing the particle size of coarse materials.

5. The Disintegrator

It works on the principle of impact and grinding.

The disintegrator consists of a drum shaped chamber made of steel. In the chamber, there are four steel beaters fixed to a disc through which passes a shaft which rotates at a high speed upto 5000 to 7000 r.p.m. The lower part of the chamber is fitted with a desired number sieve which can be easily attached or detached. A hopper is attached at the upper surface of the chamber.

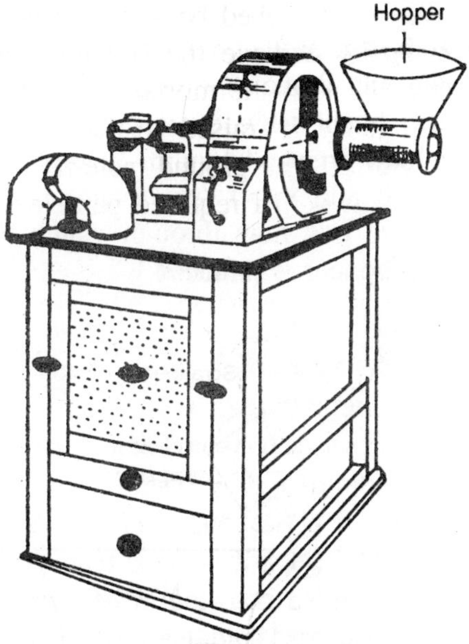

Fig. 5.7 Disintegrator

The drug to be comminuted is fed into the chamber through the hopper where it is broken by the direct blow of the beaters and by the impact of the material which is thrown with a great force against the surface of the chamber. The reduced particles pass through the sieve of desired size.

Advantages

Now a days the disintegrators have become very popular because they can be used for reducing the particle size of all kinds of materials. It has got the following advantages :

1. They can be used for powdering very hard drugs but to avoid jamming of the beaters the drug in moderately small pieces and in dry conditions should be used.
2. They are used for powdering crude vegetable drugs.
3. They can be used for milling the ointments and for mixing the powdered ingredients.

6. Bohr Stone Mill

It works on the principle of crushing and shearing.

Bohr stone mill is known by the name because two heavy stones are used in this mill. They are flat in nature and are placed horizontally one above the other with a suitable adjusting device in-between them. Both the stones have small furrows on them which help in grinding the material. Generally the lower stone is fixed and upper one rotates. In the centre of the upper stone there is a hole through which the material is fed. To this hole a hopper is attached.

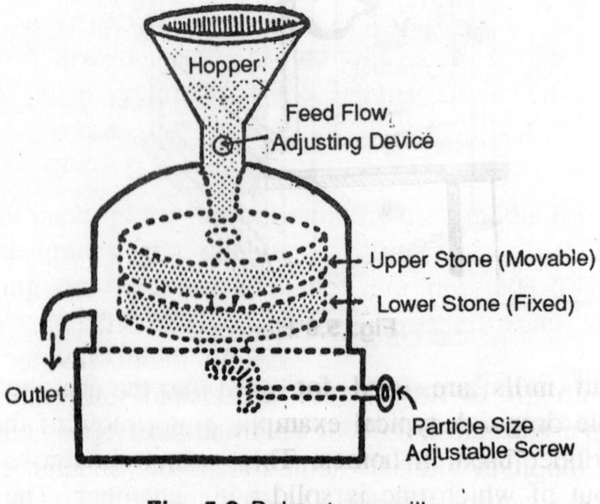

Fig. 5.8 Bohr stone mill

The material to be ground is placed in the hopper from where it is supplied in-between the two stones. Due to the heavy weight of upper stone and friction caused by the surfaces of two stones the material is reduced to fine particles. The fineness can be adjusted by adjusting the speed of upper stone and by controlling the quantity of the material supplied in-between the stones. The powdered material is collected in a container through the outlet.

Advantages

1. They can be used for making coarse or moderately fine powder.
2. Large quantities of a drug can be powdered at a time.

7. *Hand Mill*

It works on the principle of grinding.

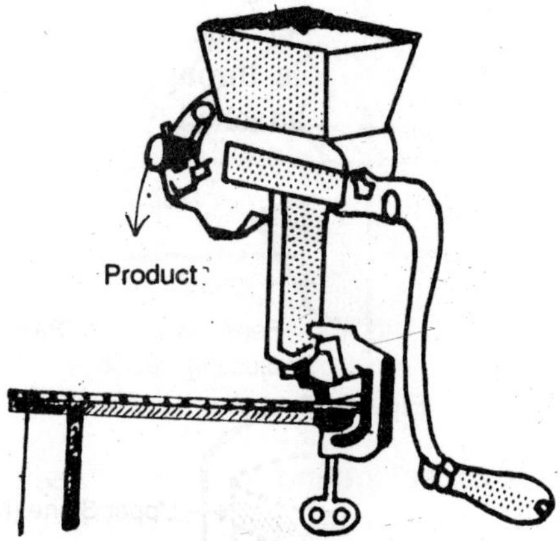

Fig. 5.9 Hand mill

Hand mills are used for grinding small quantities of vegetable drugs. A typical example of this type of mill is the hand grinder used in homes. The hand mill consists of two cones out of which one is solid and the other is hollow, the adjacent surfaces of which are toothed or corrugated. These two cones provide the grinding surface. The solid cone fits into the hollow cone which are attached to a shaft. The material to be ground is put into the machine through a hopper. By turning the handle fitted externally, the solid cone revolves by which the material is ground in small particles. The gap between the two cones can be adjusted with the help of a thumb screw fitted externally.

8. *Colloid Mill*

It works on the principle of shearing.

A colloid mill consists of a conical rotor and a stator. The gap between them can be adjusted from 0.005 to 0.075 cms. The rotor is connected to a high speed motor which can revolve at a speed of 3000 to 20000 r.p.m.

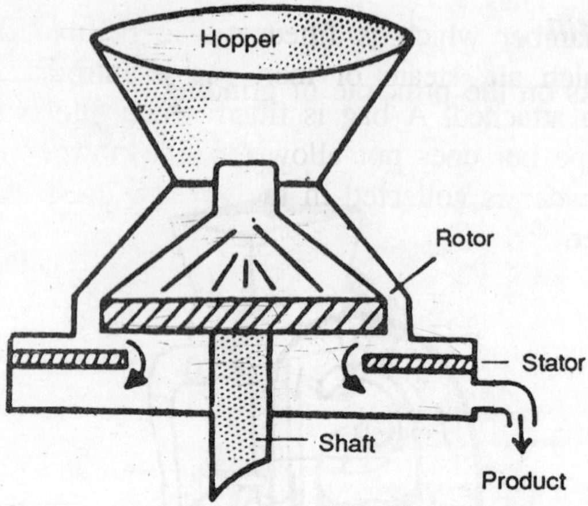

Fig. 5.10 Colloid mill

The material to be ground is already reduced to as fine particles as possible to avoid damage to the colloid mill. The reduced material is then fed into the machine through a hopper, which is thrown outward by centrifugal action. As the material passes through a narrow gap between the rotor and stator its size is reduced. The fine particles are collected from the out let in a container.

Advantages

1. Products with particle size less than one micron can be obtained with colloid mill.
2. Size reduction is always carried out in the presence of a liquid.
3. They are useful for preparing pharmaceutical suspensions, emulsions, lotions, ointments and creams.

9. Fluid Energy Mill

This mill is based on the simple principle that when two objects strike with each other with sufficient force, one or both of them break into small pieces. Thus they are broken by interparticular attrition.

These mills are also known as jet mills or micronizers which do not have any moving part. They consist of a hollow grinding chamber which is fitted with a number of nozzles through which air, steam or inert gas is introduced, a feed inlet is also attached. A bag is fitted which allows the air or gas to escape but does not allow the fine powder to go out, the fine powder is collected in the cyclone collector fitted in the chamber.

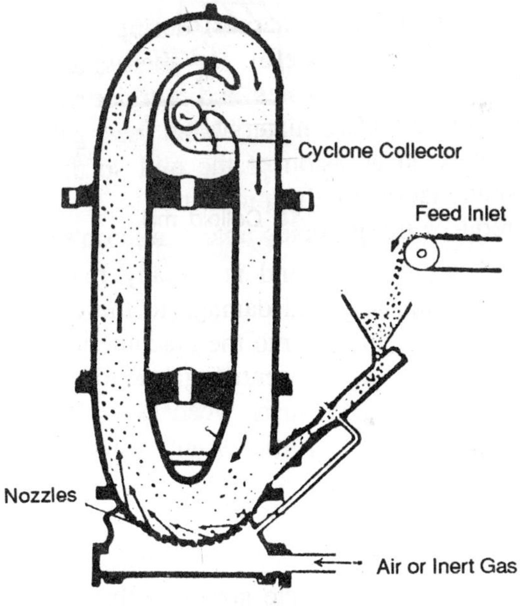

Fig. 5.11 Fluid energy mill

Pre-grinded material in the form of coarse particles are fed into the grinding chamber through the feed inlet. The elastic fluids like air, steam or an inert gas is introduced under very high pressure into the chamber through the nozzles which causes the material to circulate at high speed. The violent impact between the particles and particles, and the walls of the chamber breaks the particles into very small particles. As a result of centrifugal force the large size particles move to the outer grinding zone where they are further exposed to the attrition action. Fine particles move towards the centre of the chamber along with the exhaust gas from where they are collected in a cyclone collector.

Fluid energy mills are available in different sizes from 5 cm to 1 m in diameter, which can grind upto 2000 kg per hour depending on their size and model.

Advantages

1. These mills do not have any moving part in the grinding area.
2. Since no heat is generated during grinding therefore these mills are useful for thermolabile substances like vitamins, enzymes and antibiotics.
3. For very sensitive materials an inert gas can be used.
4. There is no abrasion of the mill so there will be no contamination of the product.
5. It reduces the particles upto 5 micron or less.

6
Size Separation

In pharmaceutical industry the control of particles size and size range is of great importance. Though various types of machines are used for size reduction but it is not necessary that they will produce the desired size particles and of uniform size. Therefore sometimes it becomes necessary to classify the powders in different grades. There are a large number of methods by which grading of powders can be done but sieving is generally used.

6.1 Sieving/sifting

Sieving or sifting is a process by which different grades of powders are separated from each other. In the laboratory different grades of sieves are used for sifting the powders and for preparing the granules of required particle size. After comminuting any material it is passed through a specific grade sieve to get the required size particles. The bigger particles are returned to the machine for regrinding. After final grinding and sieving, the material which does not pass through the sieve is known as "tailing" which should never be rejected because they may contain the medicinally active constituents. The tailing may be added to the next batch of the drug to be ground.

The ordinary sieves used in pharmacy consist of a circular frame made up of wood or metal which is fitted with a wire-cloth made of copper alloys, stainless steel, hair, silk, nylon or terylene, having specific diameter of the wire. Each sieve is given a definite number which indicates the number of meshes of standard diameter present in a length of 2.54 cm or 1 inch. The number mentioned for the sieve is the number of meshes and not the number of wires. Thus a No. 10 sieve has 10 meshes in 2.54 cm in each direction but if there are 10 wires than the number of meshes will be only 9. Since the wires occupies a sufficient space, hence the effective sifting area of apertures in a No. 10 sieve is only 44%.

6.2 Grading of powders

According to pharmacopoeia the powders can be specified into five grades depending on the size of the mesh of the sieve through which the powder can pass.

(i) Coarse powder (10/44) A coarse powder is that powder, all the particles of which pass through a No. 10 sieve and not more than 40% pass through a No. 44 sieve.

(ii) Moderately coarse powder (22/60) A moderately coarse powder is that powder, all the particles of which pass through a No. 22 sieve and not more than 40% pass through a No. 60 sieve.

(iii) Moderately fine powder (44/85) A moderately fine powder is that powder, all the particles of which pass through a No. 44 sieve and not more than 40% pass through a No. 85 sieve.

(iv) Very fine powder (120) A very fine powder is that powder, all the particles of which pass through a No. 120 sieve.

When a drug is reduced in size, particles with different sizes are produced. It is easy to get fine powder rather than coarse powder because material can be subjected to continuous grinding until fine powder is obtained. Hence the pharmacopoeia prescribes an upper and lower limit for the first three grades of coarse powders, that is why two sieves are used at a time which requires that all the particles pass through a specified number of sieve and not more than 40% pass through a finer sieve (represented as 10/44, 22/60 or 44/85). For the finer grades the pharmacopoeia prescribes only the upper limit (represented as 85 or 120).

Various grades of powders are used in different pharmaceutical processes e.g. extraction of active constituents and in the formulation of various types of dosage forms.

Water can penetrate easily into the tissues of vegetable drugs whereas alcohol (60%) tends to harden the tissues of vegetable drugs hence penetration by it is slower therefore drugs required to be extracted with alcohol should be subjected to higher degree of comminution than with aqueous solvents. Similarly drugs with softer tissues may be reduced to coarse powder whereas hard drugs should be reduced to a more finer state.

For the formulation of preparations meant for external application to the skin e.g. ointments, pastes, creams, lotions, liniments, dusting powders etc. and for ophthalmic preparations very fine powder should be used to avoid irritation due to the presence of gritty particles. For oral preparations like suspensions, powders, tablets, capsules fine powder should be used because the rate of absorption of a drug depends on the particle size, smaller the particle size quicker will be the rate of absorption. If sustained action of a drug is to be produced then large size particles will be used.

6.3 Particle size analysis

There are a large number of methods by which particle size of powders can be analysed but sieving and sedimentation methods are commonly used.

While carrying out the tests it is necessary to take a sample which should represent whole of the product. Sample should not be taken from top of the container because separation may have taken place during transport therefore preliminary mixing of the contents of the container should be done. When a number of containers are there any single container may not be typical to represent whole of the batch therefore statistical methods may be used for taking the sample, but special sampling techniques are also available.

(a) Sieving/Sifting :

Sieving is the most widely used method for measuring

particle size distribution because it is inexpensive, simple and rapid with little variation between operators.

In the sieving process the powder is passed over a perforated screen which is shaken. The particles smaller than the mesh size will pass through the sieve and oversize particles will be retained on the sieve. To obtain a distribution of particle size it is necessary to carry out a series of tests with sieves of different sizes which are arranged simultaneously one above the other and fit into each other in a tier the coarsest sieve is placed on top followed by other sieves in increasing order of their mesh numbers. The powder under test is kept in the top sieve and made to pass through a series of sieves which are shaken mechanically with gyratory (rotary movement of small amplitude) and vibratory movements to spread the material over whole of the mesh. This apparatus is useful in obtaining size analysis data under controlled conditions. The length of time and force of vibration to which the sample will be subjected is predetermined. During the vibration of sieves a fraction of powder will be retained on each sieve while other fraction will pass through the sieves. After shaking for required period of time the machine is stopped and for the purpose of analysis the weight of each fraction is determined and the percentage calculated.

With sieving method it is difficult to obtain correct results due to the reasons that :

1. Overloading of sieves may result in errors.
2. If insufficient time for shaking is allowed it may not give correct results.
3. Due to electrostatic attraction between particles the aggregates may be formed which will not pass through the sieve.
4. Due to humidity, the hygroscopic powders may lead to aggregation.
5. Particle shape has a great influence. The particles with spherical shape pass the mesh without any difficulty whereas plate like or long fibrous particles will have to be tilted into an upright position to pass the mesh.

Results of sieve analysis are best presented in the form of a cumulative oversize curve or as a histogram, since there is a wide difference in particle size range therefore size distribution curve cannot be plotted. The convenient method is to use semi-log graph paper whereby the particle size is plotted on the logarithmic scale and the proportion of material passing through the sieve is plotted on the arithmetic scale.

(b) Sedimentation methods

Sedimentation methods are based on the measurement of the rate at which particles of the powder settle out from a liquid in which they have been dispersed. This technique is widely used and can be extended to sizes of about 0.5 µm (micrometer) under special circumstances by using a centrifuge to accelerate the settlement. This method is based on the dependence of the rate of sedimentation of the particles on their size as expressed by Stoke's equation

$$de = \sqrt{\frac{18\eta}{(\rho - \rho_o)g} \frac{x}{t}}$$

Where

de = effective or Stoke's diameter

η = viscosity of the dispersion liquid in poises

x/t = rate of sedimentation or distance of fall x in time t

g = gravitational constant

ρ = density of the particles

ρ_o = density of the medium

This equation applies strictly only to dilute dispersions where the concentration of the solid does not exceed 2 percent (w/w).

The simplest method of incremental particle size analysis is the pipette method which is also known as Andreasen method. The apparatus used for this purpose is known as Andreasen apparatus which consists of a tall vessel called sedimentation vessel having capacity of 500 ml. The vessel is fitted with ground glass joint through which a 10 ml pipette fitted with two-way stopcock for draining sample is passed.

A 1 percent suspension of the powder is prepared in a suitable liquid medium which is then placed in the sedimentation vessel. As measured by the pipette 10 ml samples are withdrawn at specified intervals of time from a specified depth below the surface without disturbing the suspension. The samples are dried and the residues are weighed. As the sizes of the particles are not uniform, the particles settle at different rates. The larger particles settle at a faster rate and fall below the pipette tip sooner than the smaller particles; thus each sample withdrawn has a lower concentration and contains particles of smaller diameter than the previous sample.

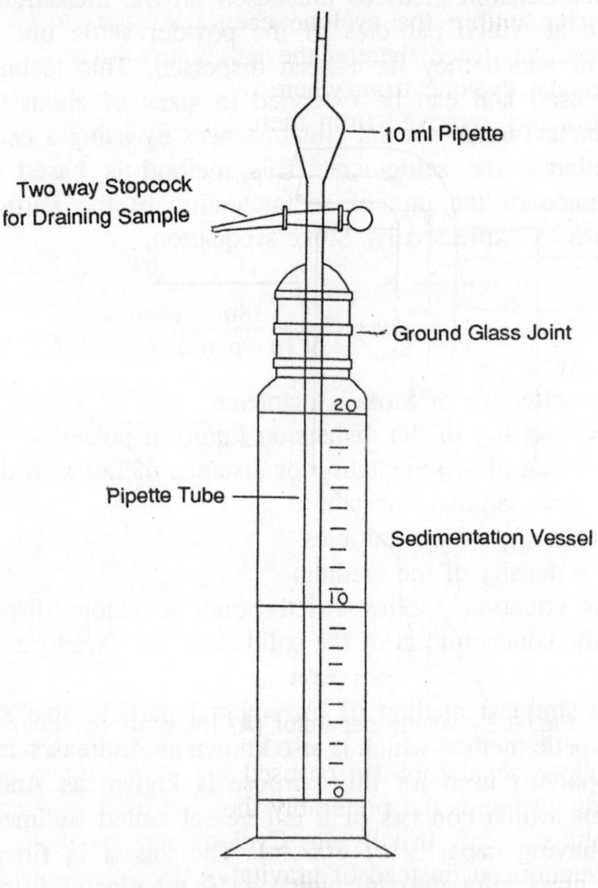

Fig. 6.1 Andreasen apparatus

From the weights of the dried samples the percentage of the initial suspension is calculated for particles having sizes smaller than the size calculated by Stoke's equation for that time.

Cyclone separator

It consists of a cylindrical vessel with a conical base. In the upper part the vessel is fitted with a tangential inlet and a fluid outlet; and at the base it is fitted with solids outlet. The suspension is introduced tangentially at a high speed so that a rotary movement takes place inside the vessel and the fluid is removed by the fluid outlet fitted at the top. The rotary movements within the cyclone causes the particles to move by centrifugal force thereby the solids are thrown out to the walls of the cyclone from where they fall to the conical base and ultimately removed from there through the solids outlet.

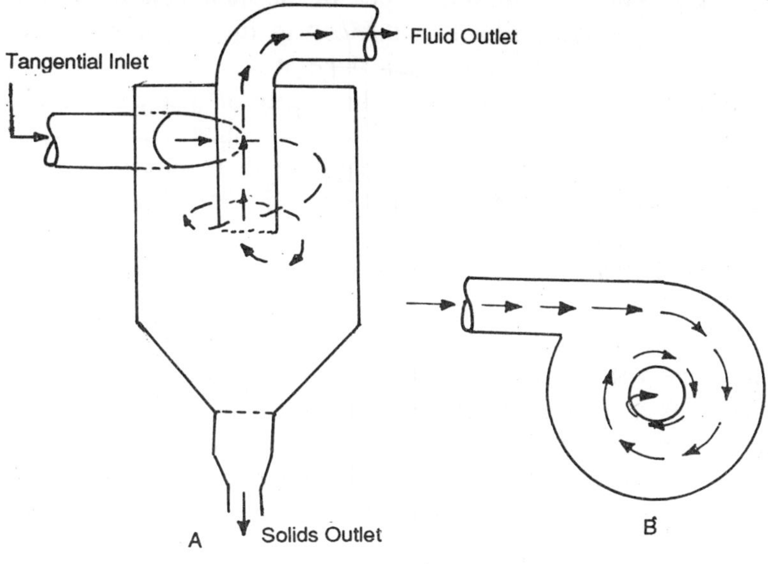

Fig. 6.2 Cyclone separator **(A)** Elevation **(B)** Plan

Cyclone separators can be used for separating suspensions of solids in liquids but preferably they are used for suspension of a solid in a gas, usually air. Cyclone separator is a form of sedimentation but instead of gravitational force the centrifugal force is used. Hence depending on the velocity of the fluid all particles can be separated with this cyclone or only the coarse particles can be removed and the fine particles are allowed to be carried with the fluid.

7
Mixing and Homogenisation

The process of mixing is one of the most commonly used operations in daily life. It is difficult to find a pharmaceutical product in which mixing is not done at one stage or the other during its manufacturing. A wide variety of materials such as liquids, viscous liquids, semi-solids and solids require mixing. Mixing is done not only in pharmaceutical industries but it has been widely used in food, plastic, glass, paint, paper, pesticides and fertilizer industries.

Mixing may be defined as the process in which two or more than two components in a separate or roughly mixed condition are treated in such a way so that each particle of any one ingredient lies as nearly as possible to the adjacent particles of other ingredients or components.

It is not possible to ascertain the degree of mixing for each and every product. It depends on the purpose of the product and the objective of the mixing operation.

7.1 Objects of mixing

Mixing may be done for following reasons :

1. To ensure uniformity of composition between the mixed ingredients which may be determined by taking samples from the bulk material and analysing them which should represent overall composition of the mixture.
2. To initiate or to enhance the physical or chemical

reactions e.g. diffusion, dissolution etc. Sometimes physical change also take place.

Generally mixing is carried out to obtain following types of products :

(i) When two or more than two miscible liquids are mixed together, a solution is produced known as true solution.

(ii) When two immiscible liquids are mixed in the presence of an emulsifying agent, an emulsion is produced.

(iii) When a solid is dissolved in a vehicle, a solution is obtained.

(iv) When an insoluble solid is mixed with a vehicle, a suspension is obtained.

(v) When a solid or liquid is mixed with a semisolid base, an ointment or a suppository is produced.

(vi) When two or more than two solid substances are mixed together, a powder is obtained which when filled into capsule shells is known as capsules and when compressed under heavy pressure is called tablets.

7.2 Types of Mixtures

Mixtures may be classified as follows :

1. Positive mixtures.
2. Negative mixtures.
3. Neutral mixtures.

1. Positive Mixtures

These types of mixtures are formed when two or more than two gases or miscible liquids are mixed together by means of diffusion process. In this case no energy is required provided the time allowed for solution formation is sufficient. Generally, these types of materials do not create any problem in mixing.

2. Negative Mixtures

These types of mixtures are formed when insoluble solids are mixed with a vehicle to form a suspension or when two immiscible liquids are mixed to form an emulsion. These mixtures are more difficult to prepare and require a higher degree of mixing with external force. The components of these mixtures separate out unless they are continuously stirred.

3. Neutral Mixtures

Many pharmaceutical products such as pastes, ointments and mixed powders are the examples of neutral mixtures. They are static in their behaviour. The components of such products do not have any tendency to mix spontaneously but once mixed, they do not separate out easily.

7.3 Mechanism of Mixing

In all types of mixers, mixing is achieved by applying one or more of the following mechanisms.

(i) Convective mixing During convective mixing transfer of groups of particles in bulk take place from one part of powder bed to another.

(ii) Shear mixing During shear mixing, shear forces are created within the mass of the material by using agitator arm or a blast of air.

(iii) Diffusive mixing During this mixing, the materials are tilted so that the gravitational forces cause the upper layers to slip and diffusion of individual particles take place over newly developed surfaces.

7.4 Rate of Mixing

Generally speaking mixing is the process of achieving uniform randomness which on subdivision to individual doses contains the correct proportions of each component which depends on the amount of mixing done. In the early stages of mixing, the rate of mixing is very fast because the mixing particles change their path of circulation quickly and find themselves in different environment whereas at the end of the process rate of mixing reaches to almost zero because the particles do not find different environment.

7.5 Liquid Mixing

Liquid mixing may be divided into following two subgroups:

(a) Mixing of liquids and liquids
  - (i) Mixing of two miscible liquids
  - (ii) Mixing of two immiscible liquids

(b) Mixing of liquids and solids
  - (i) Mixing of liquids and soluble solids
  - (ii) Mixing of liquids and insoluble solids.

(a) (i) *Mixing of two miscible liquids* (Homogeneous mixtures e.g. solutions) : Mixing of two miscible liquids is quite easy and occur by diffusion. Such type of mixing does not create any problem. Simple shaking or stirring is enough but if the liquids are not readily miscible or if they have very different viscosities then electric stirrer may be used.

(a) (ii) *Mixing of two immiscible liquids* (Heterogeneous mixtures e.g. emulsions)

When two immiscible liquids are mixed together in the presence of an emulsifying agent an emulsion is produced. For the production of a stable emulsion, the mixing must be very efficient i.e. continuous without ceasing because the components tend to separate out if continuous work is not applied on them.

Mixing Occurs in two Stages

(i) Localized mixing in which shear is applied to the particles of the liquid.

(ii) A general movement sufficient to take all the particles of the materials through the shearing zone so as to produce a uniform product.

On small scale, for the preparation of emulsions, a pestle and mortar is quite suitable. Here shear forces are produced between the flat head of the pestle and the flat bottom of the mortar whereas a general movement is produced by continuous movement of the pestle along the sides of the mortar by which the sticking material to the sides is returned to the bottom of the mortar.

Generally emulsions are prepared in two stages (i) Primary emulsion (ii) Secondary emulsion.

In the primary stage the two immiscible liquids are triturated with an emulsifying agent to get a primary emulsion which is further diluted by adding more of vehicle. After the preparation of an emulsion which is coarse is nature may be passed through a homogenizer to get a homogeneous emulsion of desired particle size.

(b) (i) *Mixing of liquids and soluble solids* (Homogeneous mixtures e.g. solutions)

In this case soluble solids are dissolved in a suitable liquid by means of stirring. It is a physical change i.e. a soluble solid is converted to a solution.

(b) (ii) *Mixing of liquids and insoluble solids* (Heterogeneous mixtures e.g. suspensions)

When insoluble solids are mixed with a vehicle a suspension is produced which is an unstable system. The ingredients of a suspension separate out when allowed to stand for sometime. Therefore to get a good suspension a suitable suspending agent should be used. On small scale, suspensions may be prepared in a pestle and mortar.

7.6 Liquid Mixers

A number of equipments e.g. shaker mixers, propeller mixers, turbine mixers and paddle mixer are used for liquid mixing but out of these propeller mixers are most widely used.

(i) Shaker mixers In these mixers, the material present in the containers is agitated either by an oscillatory or by a rotary movement. The former is applicable for small scale work whereas the latter is applicable for large scale work i.e. for rotating the large vessels similarly as that of ball mills. Shaker mixers have limited use in industries.

(ii) Propeller mixers Propeller mixers are the most widely used form of mixers for liquids of low viscosity. They are not suitable for viscous liquids like glycerin, liquid paraffin, castor oil etc. The size of the propeller is very small as compared to the size of the container. It rotates at a very high speed i.e. upto 8000 revolutions per minute due to which mixing is done in a short time.

Sometimes the high speed of the propeller may lead to undesirable vortex formation and entrapment of air (once the air bubbles are entrapped, they are difficult to remove from the product which sometimes may lead to air oxidation). This problem can be avoided in a number of ways as described below :

(i) By attaching the propeller shaft off-set from the centre (a)

(ii) By mounting the propeller at an angle (b)

(iii) By entering the propeller shaft from the side of the vessel (c)

(iv) By using a push-pull propeller (d) in which two propellers of opposite pitch are attached on the same shaft so that their rotary effects are in the opposite directions and cancel each other.

(v) By using one or more baffles, which are generally vertical strips attached to the sides of the vessel (e)

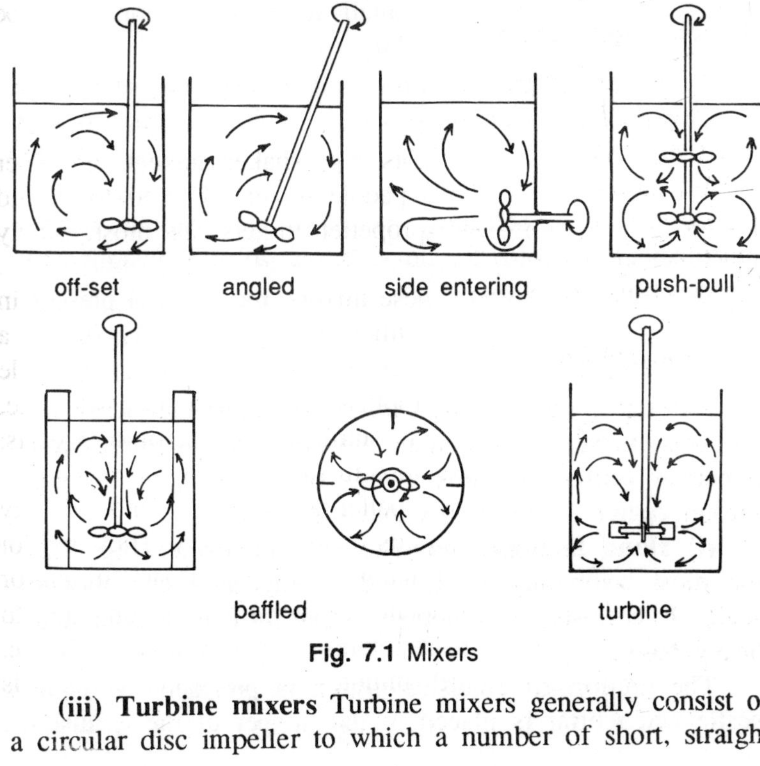

Fig. 7.1 Mixers

(iii) Turbine mixers Turbine mixers generally consist of a circular disc impeller to which a number of short, straight or curved blades are attached (Fig. f). These mixers are distinguished from propellers in that they are rotated at a lower speed than propellers and the ratio of the impeller and container diameter is also low. The former produces greater shear forces than propellers therefore they are used for mixing liquids of high viscosity and has a special application in the preparation of emulsions.

(iv) **Paddle mixers** In some of the liquid mixers, a number of paddles are used as impellers which consist of flat blades attached to a vertical shaft and rotate at a low speed of 100 r.p.m. or less. The blades have a large surface area in relation to the container in which they are employed which help them to rotate close to the walls of the container and effectively mix the viscous liquids or semi-solids. A variety of paddle mixers having different shapes and sizes, depending on the nature and viscosity of the product are available for use in industries.

7.7 Homogenization

Homogenization is the process in which a coarse emulsion is converted into a colloidal state of uniform composition by reducing the size of the particles so that each measured dose should have same composition. This process is used for the preparation of suspensions, emulsions etc. Various types of machines are used for the homogenization of emulsions which are described as follows :

7.8 Homogenizers

Homogenizers are based on the principle that when large globules in coarse emulsion are passed, under pressure, through a narrow orifice are broken into smaller globules having a greater degree of uniformity and stability.

(i) **Hand homogenizer** The Q.P. emulsifier Fig. 7.2 is the most commonly used hand homogenizer on laboratory scale. It consists of a hopper, small orifice, handle and a heavy base.

The pre-formed emulsion which is prepared by using a pestle and mortar is placed in the hopper of the emulsifier.

the emulsion is then forced to pass through a narrow orifice, by up and downward movement of the handle which reduces the size of the oil globules. this reduction in size increases with the speed of pumping.

(ii) Knewood mixer The Knewood mixer Fig. 7.3 is very effective mixing machine which has many household uses and is quite suitable for making small batches of emulsions. By this machine the mixing action is quite effective because both the beaters as well as the axis on which they are fixed rotates which produces a planetary action due to which whole of the liquid in the mixing vessel is affected and not just the central portion, which generally occurs with ordinary stirrers. Different types of beaters and whisks (e.g. coiled wire) are available with the machine which can be easily exchanged by a simple locking arrangement. In some cases the container may be fitted with a jacket so that heating or cooling of the contents may be carried out.

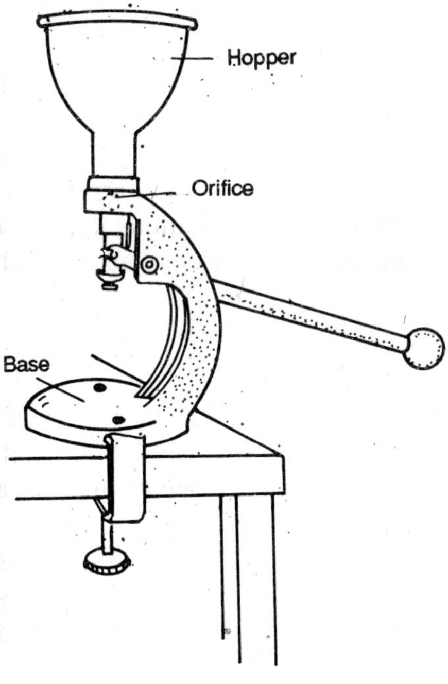

Fig. 7.2 Q.P. emulsifier

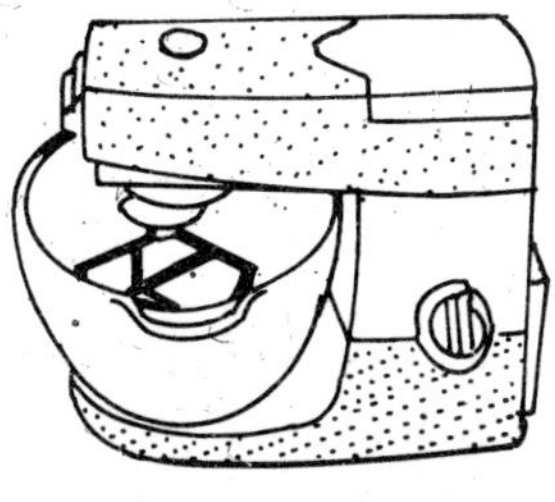

Fig. 7.3 Knewood mixer

(iii) Silverson mixer-emulsifier This machine consists of an emulsifying head to which blades are attached, surrounded by a fine mesh sieve made up of stainless steel. The emulsifying head is adjusted in such a way that it is immersed in the liquids to be emulsified. The head is rotated by means of a small motor which rotates the blades at a very high speed. The liquids to be mixed are sucked through the fine mesh into the base of the emulsifying head where they are subjected to vigorous mixing by high speed rotation of the blades. The mixed material is then expelled with a great force through the sieve band. This sucking in and forcing out of the liquid continuously goes on which sets up a pattern of circulation. In this way whole of the liquids to be mixed are made to pass repeatedly through the emulsifying head by which the large size globules are effectively reduced to small size globules. Various sizes of Silverson mixers are available which can mix a batch of liquids varying from 9 litres to 9000 litres. If necessary, the mixing vessel may be surrounded by a jacket so that the process can be carried out at desired temperatures.

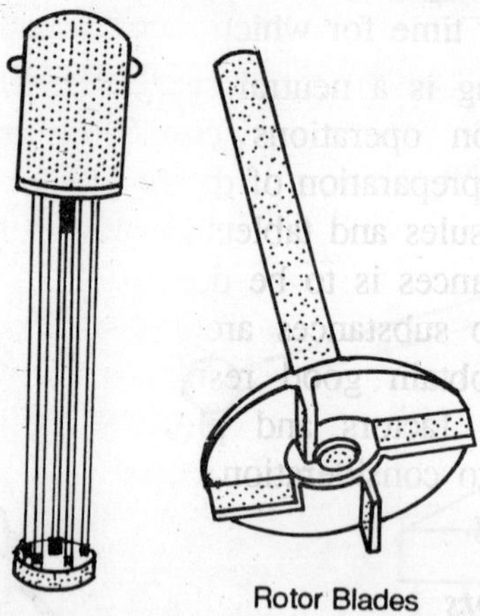

Fig. 7.4 Silverson mixer emulsifier

(iv) Ultrasonic emulsifiers Ultrasonic emulsifier works on the principle that when a liquid is subjected to ultrasonic vibrations, alternate regions of compression and rarefaction are produced which leads to the formation of cavities in the rarefaction region. Later on these cavities collapse with a great force which produces emulsification of immiscible liquids. These devices are useful only for liquids of low viscosity, moreover, they are not practicable for large scale production of emulsions.

(v) Colloid mills Colloid mills are useful for the production of colloidal dispersions and are quite suitable for the preparation of emulsions. Unlike other mixers, a continuous production can be carried out with colloid mills.

Detailed discussion of colloid mill is done in the chapter of size reduction.

7.9. Powder Mixing

Powder mixing is a process in which two or more than two solid substances are intermingled in a mixer by continuous movement of the particles. Mainly, the object of mixing operation is to produce a bulk mixture which when divided into different doses, every unit of dose must contain the correct proportion of each ingredient. The degree of mixing will increase with the length of time for which mixing is done.

Powder mixing is a neutral type of mixing. It is one of the most common operations employed in pharmaceutical industries for the preparation of different types of formulations e.g. powders, capsules and tablets. When grinding and mixing of different substances is to be done simultaneously then two or more than two substances are fed to the mill one at the same time. To obtain good results of powder mixing the following mixing factors and physical properties of drugs must be taken into consideration before undertaking any kind of powder mixing.

(a) Mixing Factors

(i) Volume The mixer must not be filled to the brim. Sufficient empty space should be provided for dilation of the bed. Overfilling of the mixer reduces the efficiency and sometimes mixing may be entirely prevented.

(ii) Mixing mechanism The mixing mechanism plays a major role in powder mixing therefore the mixer selected for the purpose must apply suitable shear forces and connective movement so that whole of the material passes through the mixing area.

(iii) **Duration of mixing** Mixing of powders must be done for optimum time for any particular situation.

(iv) **Handling of the mixed powders** After mixing the powders, they should be handled in such a way that the separation of ingredients is minimised which may be caused due to vibrations during transport, subsequent manipulation, handling etc. Therefore bulk powders should be remixed before its use.

(b) Physical Properties

(i) **Density** If the densities of mixing ingredients are different then it is quite difficult to mix them thoroughly because the heavier material moves downward through the lighter material resulting in the improper mixing of the ingredients. Therefore for uniform mixing of powders in a mixer due consideration should be given to the density of materials to be mixed.

(ii) **Particle size** Substances with different particle size are difficult to mix and may lead to segregation because the smaller particles can move downward through the spaces between the larger particles.

(iii) **Particle shape** Spherical shape of particles is ideal for mixing the powders and any deviation from this shape leads to difficulty in mixing but on the other hand, particles with irregular shapes can interlock with each other therefore chances of segregation are minimised once mixing has been done.

(iv) **Particle attraction** Some particles exert electrostatic charges due to which the particles of one powder may attract the particles of other powder leading to aggregation of particles. This effect increases as particle size decreases.

(v) **Proportions of materials to be mixed** The proportions of materials to be mixed play a very important role in powder mixing. It is easy to mix the powders if they are available in equal quantities but it is difficult to mix small quantities of powders with large quantities of other ingredients or diluents.

The general practical method for mixing such quantities is that the component present in lesser amount is mixed with an equal amount of the diluent. Then a further amount of diluent is incorporated which is almost equal to previous quantities and so on until whole of the diluent has been added. This method is followed for mixing potent substances with diluents. When more than two components are to be mixed, they should always be mixed in ascending order of their weights so as to ensure uniform mixing of the ingredients.

7.10 Mechanism of Mixing

It has been generally accepted that in all the mixers, solid mixing is achieved by a combination of one or more of the following mechanisms :

(i) Convective mixing In convective mixing transfer of groups of particles takes place from one location to another by means of blades or paddles of the machine.

(ii) Shear Mixing In shear mixing, slip planes are set up within the mass of the material.

(iii) Diffusive mixing During this mechanism, mixing occurs by "diffusion" process by random movement of particles within a powder bed and cause them to change their relative positions.

7.11 Equipment used for Mixing of Powders

The following equipment is used for powder mixing :

(i) Pestle and mortar
(ii) Spatula
(iii) Sieves
(iv) Tumbler mixers
(v) Agitator mixers

(i) By pestle and mortar Pestle and mortar is most commonly used for small scale mixing specially required in compounding of prescriptions. In this method, particle size reduction and mixing is done in a single operation. Therefore, it is particularly useful when some degree of particle size reduction as well as mixing is required.

(ii) By spatula Sometimes small quantities of powders can be mixed on a piece of paper or glazed tile with the help of a bone spatula. This method is relatively inefficient but is used when compaction produced by pestle and mortar method is undesirable.

(iii) By sieves Sieves are generally used for breaking the loose aggregates of powders in pre or post mixing operation so as to increase overall effectiveness of a blending technique. Sometimes powder may have to be passed a number of times through the sieves to get a homogeneous powder.

(iv) Tumbler mixers For large scale mixing or batch mixing of powders these mixers are used. A common type of mixer consists of metallic container which is rotated on its horizontal axis by means of a motor. The most popular mixer is the twin-shell blender "V" shape. When this is rotated the material collected in the bottom of V splits into two portions when the V is inverted. This design is quite effective because bulk transport and shear forces are enhanced. To improve agitation of the powder bed, a bar fitted with blades which rotate in the opposite direction to that of blender may be attached. Various other types of tumbler mixers e.g. cubical, double cone, Y-shaped and cylindrical are used which may be rotated on any axis.

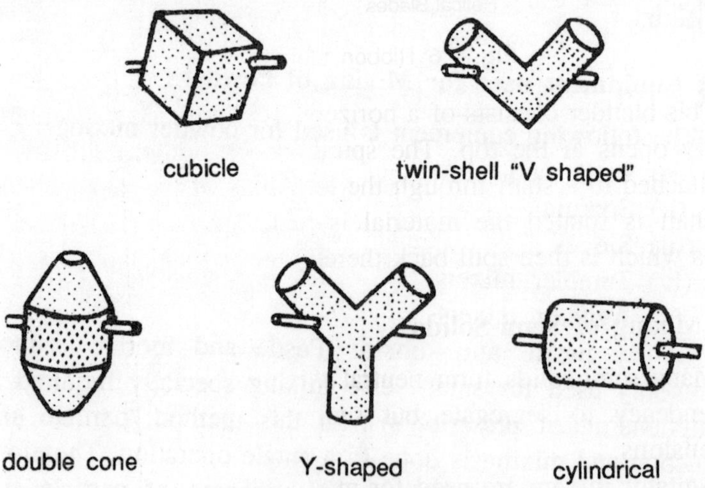

Fig. 7.5 Tumblers

The efficiency of tumbler mixers depends on the speed of rotation. If the speed of rotation is too slow it will cause sliding only i.e. at the highest position the powder will fall to the bottom and desired tumbling will not be produced. But on the other hand if rotation is too high it will produce sufficient centrifugal forces which will hold the powder along the sides of the mixer, and will not allow the powder to fall down thereby there will be no mixing. The optimum speed of a mixer is 30 to 100 r.p.m.

(v) Agitator mixers These are another type of mixers in which the container to hold the material is fixed and mixing is done by means of mixing screws, paddles or blades. They are useful for mixing powders of sticky or plastic consistency. The high shear forces set up breaks the lumps or aggregates. The most popular mixer of this type is the ribbon blender Fig. 7.6.

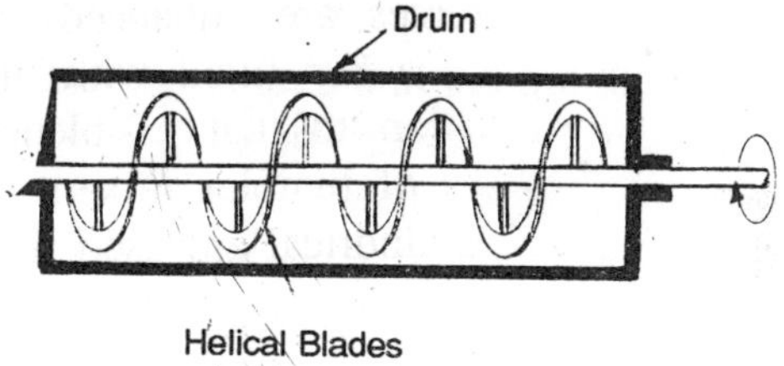

Fig. 7.6 Ribbon blender

This blender consists of a horizontal cylindrical tank which usually opens at the top. The spiral blades or helical blades are attached to a shaft through the long axis of the tank. when the shaft is rotated the material is picked up by the helical blades which is then spilt back thereby the particles are mixed.

7.12 Mixing of Semi-Solids

Many semi-solids form neutral mixture because they have no tendency to segregate but sedimentation may occur in suspensions.

Agitator mixers are used for mixing the semi-solids. They work on the same principle as that used for mixing the liquids and for powders. Planetary motion mixers designed specially for semi-solids are of heavy construction because they are to handle very thick materials. The arms of the agitator are designed in such a way that they produce pulling and kneading action and also clear whole of the material from all sides and corners of the mixing vessel.

The most commonly used mixer for mixing the semi-solids is the sigma-arm mixer. It is so named because the shape of two mixer blades used resembles the Greek letter, sigma. The two blades rotate towards each other but at different speeds. Because of heavy construction and high power of mixing, this mixer can handle products such as pill masses, tablet granulation masses, ointments and pastes. To work at high or low temperatures the vessel is enclosed in a jacket through which steam or cold water may be circulated. The planetary and sigma blade mixers are used for wet granulation and can handle 100 to 200 kg of the material. Because these mixers are fitted with motors in the range of 7 to 10 horsepower therefore can impart far greater kneading and massing action than the laboratory equipments.

The major difficulty encountered in mixing the semi-solids is the entrainment of air. This difficulty can be overcome if the mixing is done under reduced pressure but care must be taken when the mixing ingredients also contain volatile substances.

Triple roller mill

Various types of roller mills consisting of one or more rollers are commonly used but triple roller mill is preferred. It is fitted with three rollers which are composed of a hard abrasion-resistant material. They are fitted in such a way that they come in close contact with each other and rotate at different speeds. The material which come, inbetween the rollers is crushed and reduced in particle size. The reduction in particle size depends on the gap between the rollers and difference in their speeds. A typical diagram (cross section) of triple roller mill is shown in Fig. 7.7.

The material is allowed to pass through hopper A, inbetween the rollers B and C where it is reduced in size. Then the material is passed between the rollers C and D where it is further reduced in size and a smooth mixture is obtained.

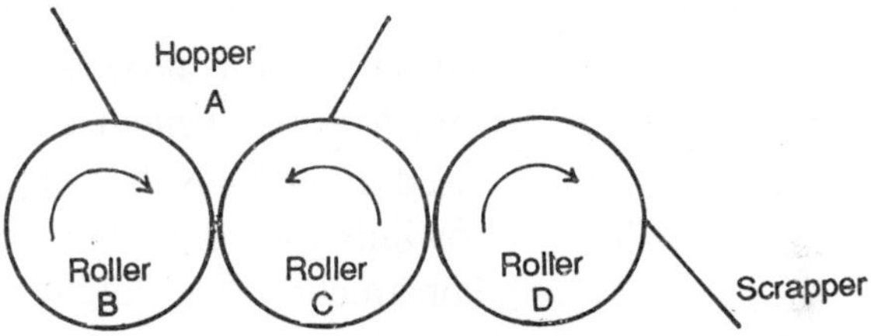

Fig 7.7 Triple roller mill

The gap between rollers C and D is usually less than the gap between B and C, After passing the material between rollers C & D the smoothened material is continuously removed from roller D by means of scraper E, from where it is collected in a receiver.

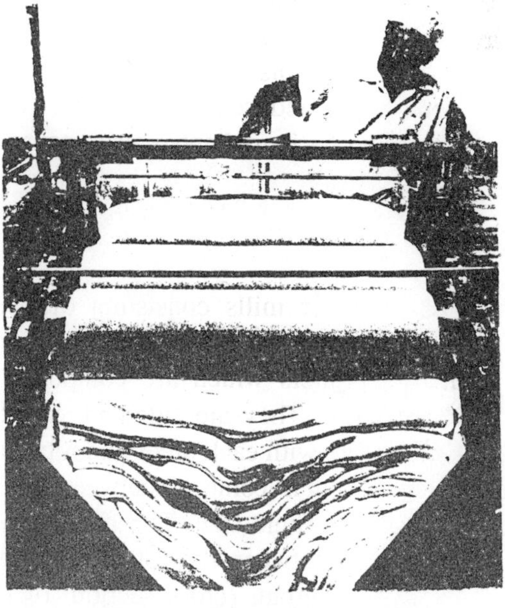

Fig 7.8 Ointment roller mill

On large scale, mechanical ointment roller mills are used to obtain an ointment of smooth and uniform texture. The preformed coarse ointments are forced to pass through moving stainless steel rollers where it is reduced in particle size and a smooth product which is uniform in composition and texture is obtained. For small scale work, small ointment mills are available.

8

Filtration and Clarification

Filtration may be defined as the process in which solids are separated from liquids by means of a porous medium which retains the solids but allows the liquid to pass through it and optically transparent liquid free from insoluble solids, colloidal hazes, or insoluble liquid drops is obtained.

The term clarification is used when the solids present in the liquid is very small and they do not exceed 1.0 per cent and filtrate is the required product.

The suspension of solids and liquids to be filtered is known as feed or slurry and the porous medium through which the slurry is forced to pass is called filter medium, the solids collected on the filter medium is referred to as filter cake and clear liquid which passes through the filter is called filtrate. When solids collected on the filter medium is the desired product then the process is known as cake filtration.

The mechanism of filtration is based on two operations that is

(i) the flow of solids is resisted by the filter medium while the liquid is allowed to pass.

(ii) as the filtration proceeds the retention of solids on the filter media goes on increasing which acts as a secondary and sometimes more efficient filtering medium.

Factors Affecting Rate of Filtration

The factors which affect the rate of filtration of any liquid is expressed by Darcy's law which is stated as under :

$$\frac{dV}{dt} = \frac{KA\,\Delta P}{\eta l}$$

where V = volume of filtrate

t = time of filtration

K = constant for the filter medium and filter cake.

A = area of filter medium

ΔP = pressure difference above the filter medium and below the filter medium i.e. on the filtrate.

η = viscosity of the filtrate.

l = thickness of the filter bed i.e. thickness of the filter cake and filter medium.

The above law represents the rate of flow through the capillaries of the filter medium and filter cake. From the above equation it is clear that the rate of filtration depends upon a number of factors and not only the liquid which is undergoing filtration.

The factors which govern the rate of filtration are as follows:

1. Area of Filter Surface

Rate of filtration is directly proportional to the area of filter surface. Greater the filtering surface greater will be the rate of filtration e.g. with the use of pleated filter paper filtration is increased.

2. Particle Size of the Solids to be Removed

Rate of filtration is directly proportional to the particle size of the solids to be removed.

3. Pore Size of the Filter Media

Rate of filtration is directly proportional to the pore size of the filter media.

4. The Resistance of the Filter Cake and Filter Media

The rate of flow will be greatest at the beginning of the process because there is minimum resistance but as the process proceeds the filter cake is formed which goes on increasing and adding thickness to the cake which slows down the rate of filtration but this cake also acts as a secondary filter medium.

5. Viscosity of the Liquid to be filtered

The rate of filtration is inversely proportional to the viscosity of the liquid to be filtered. Liquids with low viscosity get filtered quickly whereas thick liquids get filtered slowly. The rate of filtration of such liquids can be increased by applying pressure on the viscous liquids or by increasing the temperature of liquid to be filtered.

6. Temperature

Increased temperature reduces the viscosity of thick liquids such as syrup, glycerin, liquid paraffin etc. thus they can be filtered quickly.

In some cases filter presses are so constructed that they can be maintained at high temperatures through which viscous liquids are to be filtered.

7. Pressure Difference Across the Filter

The rate of filtration is directly proportional to the pressure difference across the filter bed. The rate of filtration can be increased by increasing the pressure on the liquid to be filtered (cake filtration) or by reducing the pressure under the filter media i.e. in the receiver (vacuum filtration).

8.1 Filter Media

The surface or medium upon which solids are retained in the process of filtration is known as filter media.

An ideal filter media should have the following properties:

(i) It should be chemically inert.
(ii) It should have high retention power for the solids but should allow the maximum passage of the liquids.
(iii) It should have sufficient mechanical strength to withstand filtration pressure.
(iv) It should absorb negligible amounts of dissolved material.

(v) It should be resistant to the corrosive action of the liquid.

While selecting the filter media the following factors must be taken into consideration.

(i) Size of the particles to be filtered.
(ii) Amount of the liquid to be filtered.
(iii) Nature of the product to be filtered i.e. a solution, suspension or a viscous preparation.
(iv) Purpose of filtration i.e. only to get clear preparation or to get a clear sterile preparation.

There are a wide range of filter media used for pharmaceutical processes which are discussed below :

1. Filter Paper

Filter paper is the most commonly used media for filtration. Different grades and qualities of filter paper are available. Depending on the pore size they are referred to as coarse, medium and fine. Only high quality filter paper should be used to get maximum filtering efficiency.

Though filter papers are widely used as filter media but they shed very fine particles to the filtrate moreover they have the tendency to absorb small quantity of liquid.

2. Woven Materials

Woven materials such as cloth made from cotton, silk, wool, rayon, nylon or glass act as filter media. Fine muslin made from cotton is widely used for removing very coarse particles but it can shed particles to the filtrate; has a great tendency to absorb liquid and can be destroyed by certain chemicals. Nylon cloth is also used for coarse filtration. It is superior to cotton cloth for pharmaceutical use in that the nylon is not affected by mold, fungus or bacteria and has negligible absorption properties. Nylon cloth is extremely strong as compared to cotton cloth. Due to above mentioned reasons synthetic cloth is preferred for filtration in pharmaceutical processes.

Woven wire cloth particularly made from stainless steel is quite durable, long lasting and easily cleaned which can be reused. They are resistant to chemicals and can be easily sterilized. Wire cloth filter media afford good surface for cake filtration and are generally used with filter aids.

3. Cotton wool

Cotton wool is commonly used for filtering the coarse particles. A small tuft of cotton wool is placed in the neck of the funnel and the liquid is poured over it. The cotton wool has disadvantage that small filaments are detached from it which are carried to the filtrate. This difficulty can be reduced to a minimum by using cotton wool prepared from high quality cotton with long staple and by wetting the cotton with the menstruum before inserting it in the funnel.

4. Glass Wool

Glass wool is used for filtering highly corrosive chemicals such as strong acids, strong alkalies and oxidising agents e.g. solutions of potassium permanganate and chromic acid. Filter paper and cotton wool can't be used for filtering above mentioned substances because both these filters get destroyed. Although glass wool provides very effective filter medium but it may contaminate the filtrate with glass fibres.

5. Asbestos

Asbestos is also used for filtering the corrosive liquids. Asbestos pads are prepared by compressing shredded asbestos tightly under pressure. These pads have disadvantages in that (i) they impart alkalinity to the filtrate (ii) certain substances like alkaloids may get adsorbed on them (iii) asbestos fibres may contaminate the filtrate.

6. Kraft paper

Kraft paper is mainly used in plate and frame filters and horizontal plate filters. They offer controlled porosity, limited absorption properties and are quite cheap. White papers are preferred for pharmaceutical work. When used in large filter presses they require a support of cloth or wire mesh, to prevent rupture of the paper with pressure.

7. Sintered Glass

Sintered glass filters consists of pyrex glass powdered and sifted to produce granules of uniform size which are then heated to fuse them. The interstices between the particles form a connective system through which liquid can pass. The sintered glass can be fused in an ordinary funnel or in a Buchner funnel for filtration under reduced pressure. Various shapes and grades of these funnels are available.

These filters are used for filtering parenteral preparations and solutions meant for eyes. They are also useful for filtering corrosive liquids and oxidizing agents. Sintered glass filters do not shed particles, do not absorb any liquid and can be easily washed for re-use. For cleaning they may be scrubbed gently with a soft brush and a stream of water is introduced through the reverse direction or by chemical methods.

Note : For discussion of sintered glass funnel please refer to 'Sterilization' chapter.

8. Membrane Filters

These are thin porous membranes made from cellulose esters or similar polymeric materials or from nylon, teflon or polyvinylchloride. They are mainly used for filtration of parenteral solutions or preparations meant for ophthalmic use.

Note : Please refer to 'Sterilization' chapter also.

9. Cartridge Units

Different types of filter media are also available as cartridge units. They are used for removing low percentage of solids ranging from 100 microns to less then 1 micron in size. Two types of cartidge units are available (i) surface type and (ii) depth type. The surface type cartridges are made up of porcelain or kieselguhr in the form of candles. They can be cleaned easily for reuse by backflushing. The depth type cartridges consist of fibrous media like cotton, asbestos or cellulose. These can be used only once because they are difficult to clean and they have the tendency to shed fibres.

8.2 Filter Aids

While filtering liquids containing slimy compressible materials, the filter media soon get clogged and it becomes necessary to add a material which will check this problem, such type of substances are known as filter aids.

Filter aids may be defined as the substances which when added to the liquid to be filtered, reduce the resistance of the filter cake and increase the filtration. These substances form a porous, non-compressible cake which can retain the solid particles but allow the liquid to flow through it. A concentration of 0.1 to 0.5% of filter aid is added to the preparation before filtration. They may be added directly to the suspension to be filtered or a suspension of filter aid is first prepared in a suitable liquid which is then added to the liquid to be filtered. An ideal filter aid should have the following characteristics :

(i) It should be chemically inert.
(ii) It should have low specific gravity.
(iii) It should be insoluble in the liquid to be filtered.
(iv) It should form a porous cake.
(v) It should be readily recoverable from the liquid.

The substances which are used as filter aids include kieselguhr, talc, charcoal, asbestos, paper pulp, kaolin, chalk, magnesium carbonate and bentonite.

8.3 Methods and Equipment Required for Filtration

The selection of a method and equipment required for filtration of a liquid depends on the nature of the material and quantity to be filtered as well as the object of the operation. Various types of equipment used for filtration are discussed below :

1. Filter Funnels

Funnels are conical shaped devices which help in pouring the liquids in narrow mouth containers. They are widely used for supporting the filter media. Funnels are generally made up of glass, polythene, copper, aluminium, stainless steel or any other suitable metal. Glass funnels made from neutral glass are most commonly used for small scale filtration.

Generally funnels with plane surface are used but they may be fluted, grooved or ribbed to increase the downward flow of the filtrate. A white filter paper of suitable pore size is selected which is folded in such a way that it fits in the funnel. To increase the rate of filtration a pleated filter paper is used by which effective filtration surface will be increased to a considerable extent. Polythene funnels are not suitable for corrosive substances.

2. Buchner Funnels

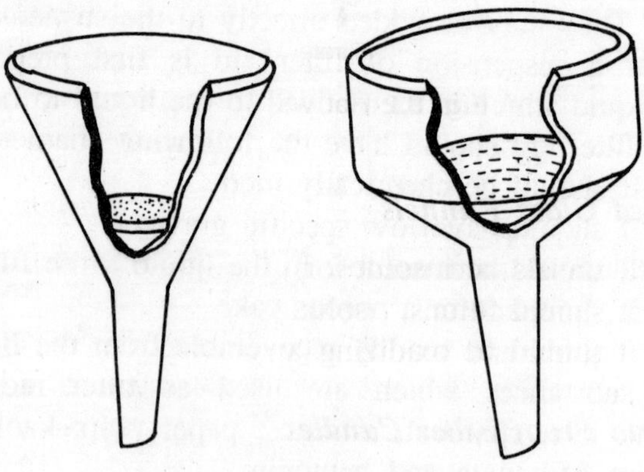

Fig. 8.1 Buchner funnels

Buchner funnels also known as Hirsch funnels are made up of porcelain which are modified in such a way that a disc of filter paper is supported on a perforated plate. These funnels are especially used for filtration under reduced pressure. They are also used for washing the precipitates.

3. Hot Water Funnels

Hot water funnels or Jacketed funnels are double walled funnels made up of a metal. Viscous substances such as liquid paraffin, glycerin, castor oil and fatty substances like wool fat, bees wax, soft paraffin, hard paraffin, ointments and creams etc. are difficult to filter at ordinary temperature but they can be filtered easily if the temperature of the funnel is maintained at a higher level throughout the process which is done by using hot water funnels. Boiling water or steam is circulated in the jacketed funnel.

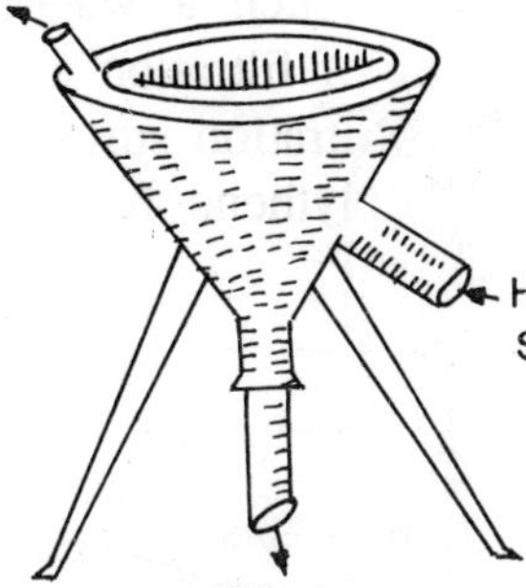

Fig. 8.2 Hot water funnel

4. Sintered Glass Funnels

These funnels are used for filtering parenteral products, ophthalmic preparations, solutions of potent substances, corrosive liquids and oxidizing agents.

5. Bacteria Proof Filter Candles

6. Millipore Filters

7. Membrane Filters

Note : For detailed discussion of sintered glass funnels, bacteria proof filters, millipore filters and membrane filters please refer to 'Sterilization' chapter.

8. Filter Leaf

Filter leaf consists of a frame in which a drainage screen or a grooved plate is enclosed. The whole unit is covered with a cloth which acts as a filter media. The inside of the frame is fitted with an outlet and an attachment to connect to the vacuum pump. The frame of the filter may be of any shape i.e. round, square or rectangular.

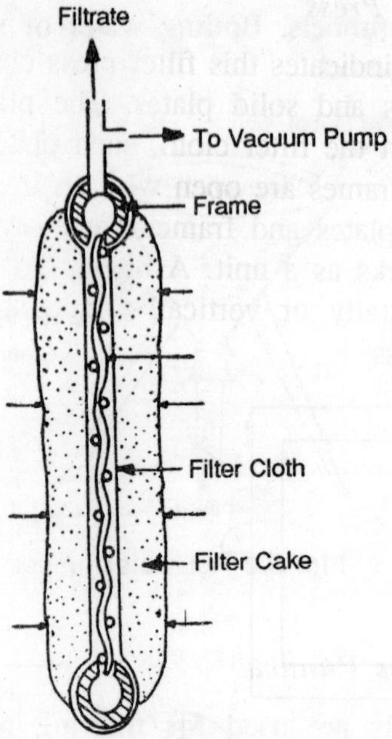

Fig. 8.3 Filter leaf

For use the filter leaf is immersed in the container having the slurry to be filtered and the vacuum system is connected to the filtrate outlet. When the vacuum will be created the filtration will start and the filtrate will go on collecting in the receiver. The cake will be deposited on the outer surface of the filter cloth which can be easily washed with water or removed by backward flow of air through the unit.

This method has the advantage that the liquid can be filtered from any vessel and deposited cake can be removed simply by washing or by blowing air in the reverse direction through the system. This is most satisfactory method if the solid contents in the liquid are not more than 5%. The labour costs involved in operating the filter leaf are also comparatively low.

9. Filter Press

Various types of filter presses are used for large scale filtration but the plate and frame press is widely used in pharmaceutical industries.

Plate and Frame Press

As the name indicates this filter press consists of a number of hollow frames and solid plates. The plates have grooved surface to support the filter cloth, each plate has an outlet for the filtrate. The frames are open with an inlet for the liquid to be filtered. The plates and frames are assembled alternatively and each set works as a unit. A number of such sets may be arranged horizontally or vertically and fixed with the outer frame of the press.

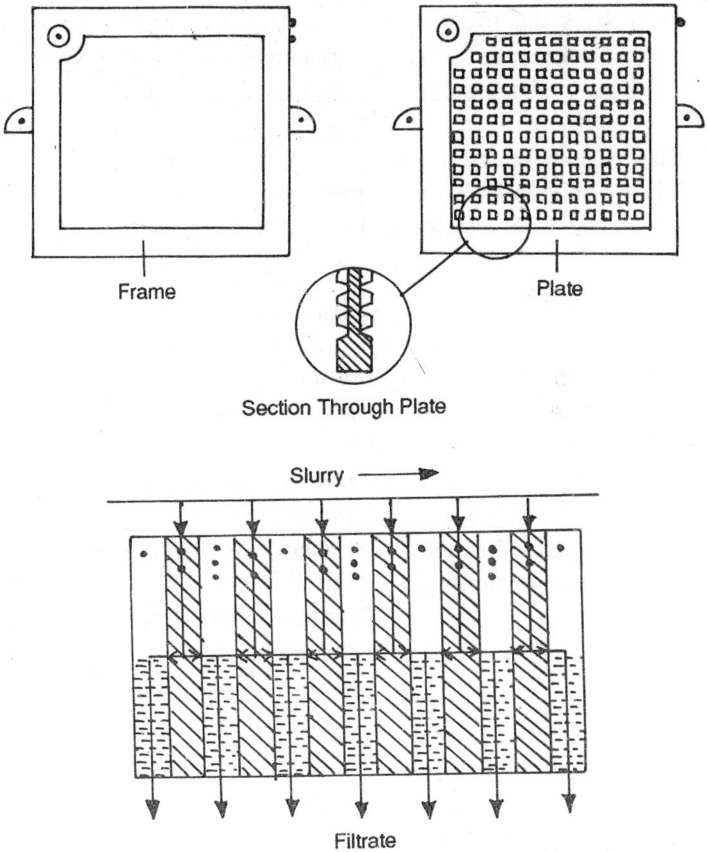

Fig. 8.4 Frame, plate and filter press showing operation

The liquid to be filtered is allowed to enter the frame under pressure, the filtrate passes through the filter medium on to the surface of the plate while the filter cake is retained in the frame. The filtrate drains out of the plate through the outlet. The operation is continued till the frame is filled with the filter cake. When the process is stopped, the filter cake is removed from the frame and the process is restarted.

Advantages

(i) The construction is very simple and a number of materials ranging from wood to stainless steel may be used for its construction.
(ii) It is the most versatile filter press because the filter media can be varied to suit a particular requirement and even bacteria proof filtration may be carried out with it.
(iii) It can be used for coarse to fine filtration.
(iv) The operation and maintenance is easy.
(v) The filter cloth can be easily replaced.

Disadvantages

(i) This filter press is for batch filtration and filtration of small quantities are not economical
(ii) The filter press is quite costly and labour cost involved in replacement of filter cloth is also high.
(iii) This press is suitable when the slurry contains less than 5% solids.
(iv) Leakage between the plates may take place through faulty assembly.

10. Rotary Filters

When the proportion of solid contents in the slurry is in the range of 15-30% and it is not possible to filter them by filter leaf or filter press then rotary drum filters are used. It is a continuous process and is used in pharmaceutical industries for large scale operation. These filters work on the principle like that of filter leaf.

Rotary drum filters consist of a perforated metal drum wrapped with filter cloth or other suitable material to act as filter medium The drum is partially immersed in the tank containing the material to be filtered, the drum is rotated at a slow speed i.e. even less than 1 rev per min; and vacuum created. As soon as the vacuum will be created the filtrate will enter into the drum through the filter medium and filter cake will be deposited on the outer surface of the filter medium. This cake is then removed by scraping with a knife just before the rotating drum repeats another cycle. The above mentioned operation continues till the slurry gets exhausted.

Advantages

(i) Since the filtration process is automatic and continuous the overall labour costs are very low.
(ii) The area of filtration is very high so a large quantity of slurry can be filtered at a time.
(iii) The thickness of filtration cake can be controlled by altering the speed of rotation of the drum.

Disadvantages

(i) This filter is very expensive.
(ii) This process cannot be used for slurries containing low percentage of solids.

11. Meta Filters

In some pharmaceutical processes where filter presses are not convenient to handle small quantities, there meta filters are used. The simplest form of metafilter consists of a grooved drainage rod on which a series of metal rings made from stainless steel are packed. The rings are of 22 mm outer dia, 15 mm inside dia. and 0.8 mm in thickness. When the rings are tightened on the drainage rod with a nut, tapered channels from 250 μm to 25 μm are formed.

This unit is placed in the vessel containing the slurry to be filtered. When the vacuum is created the liquid passes through the pack into the drainage rod and ultimately to the receiver. These filters may be fitted with a steam jacket for the filtration of very viscous liquids such as syrups or oily substances. They are also useful for the clarification of parenteral solutions. Metafilters are used as strainers for coarse particles but for finer particles a bed of some suitable material such as kieselguhr, charcoal or other filter aid is first deposited on the pack of rings on which true filter medium is supported.

12. Filtration under Reduced Pressure

On laboratory scale, filtration under reduced pressure is carried out in an apparatus consisting of a Buchner funnel, filtration flasks and a filter pump. The Buchner funnel is fitted in the filtration flask made up of specially strong glass, the side tube of which is attached to another flask to avoid the risk of 'back suction'. The second flask is connected to a filter pump. A filter paper of good quality cut to the size of Buchner funnel is placed over the perforations of the Buchner funnel and liquid to be filtered is poured over the filter paper. When vacuum is created by opening the water tap to which filter pump is attached, filtration starts at a high speed and filtrate collects in the filtration flask. This method is quite commonly used in the laboratories for filtration of liquids and for washing the precipitates in analytical work.

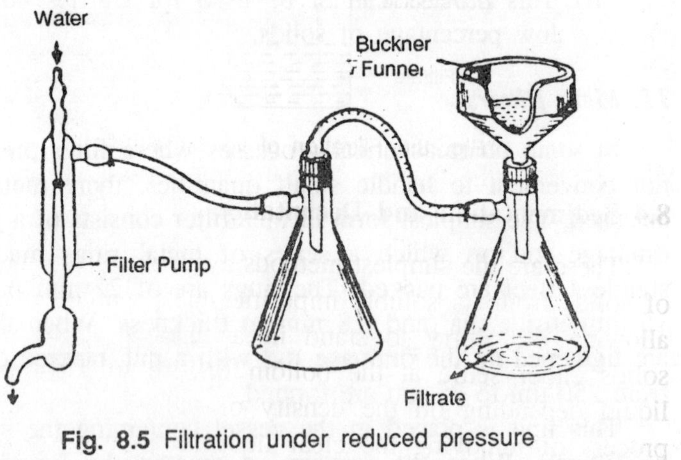

Fig. 8.5 Filtration under reduced pressure

13. Filtration of Volatile Liquids

It is not feasible to filter the volatile liquids and flammable volatile liquids by ordinary methods of filtration because of loss through evaporation and liability to explosion respectively. Therefore for filtration of such liquids the funnels must be covered and receivers must be closed and provision must be made for the air to escape from the receiver. Diagram is shown in Fig. 8.6

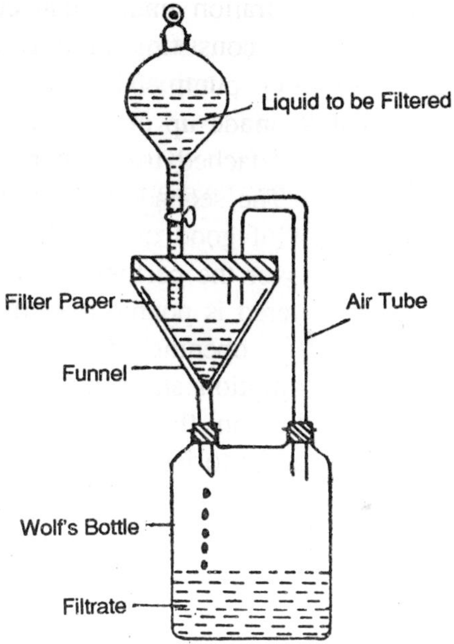

Fig. 8.6 Filtration of volatile liquids

8.4 Sedimentation and Decantation

These are the simplest methods available for the separation of solids from its soluble impurities. The method consists of allowing the slurry to stand in a suitable vessel until the solids either settle at the bottom or rise to the top of the liquid depending on the density of the solid particles. The process of removing the clear liquid from the top is called decantation and settling of solids at the bottom is known as sedimentation. The process of sedimentation can be hastened by centrifugation. These methods are used for washing the precipitates or magmas. The washing is repeated as often as necessary until the desired purity of the solids is attained.

8.5 Straining

Colation or straining is a simplest and crude method of filtration. In this process the slurry to be filtered is poured on a muslin cloth or a porous substance which will allow the liquid to pass through but will retain the solids over it. This method is generally used for separating the solid impurities from liquids. The apparatus used for straining is very simple which generally consists of a strainer medium and a support or frame for the strainer medium. The strainer medium is usually colourless cloth material such as flannel, muslin, wool and cheese cloth. The strainer medium must be washed before use.

9

Extraction and Galenicals

Extraction may be defined as the process in which the animal or plant tissues are treated with specific solvents whereby the medicinally active constituents are dissolved out, cell tissues and most of inactive or inert components remain undissolved. In pharmacy, the solvent used for extraction purposes is known as menstruum and residue left after extracting the desired constituents is known as marc.

The products obtained after extraction are impure and intended only for oral and external use. Such preparations include infusions, decoctions, tinctures, liquid extracts, semisolid extracts and powdered extracts. These types of preparations are known as galenicals after the Greek Physician Galen. Previously they were extensively used than at present. They were generally used for extemporaneous dispensing and were required to be freshly prepared.

9.1 Solvents used for the extraction of Drugs

There are a large number of solvents (menstruum) used for the extraction of drugs but the selection of a suitable solvent capable of extracting the active constituents depends upon the chemical properties of active constituents as well as the qualities of the solvent. An ideal solvent for the extraction of drugs should be cheap, physically and chemically inert, non-toxic and selective i.e. it should dissolve only the required constituents with minimum amount of the inert materials but these qualities are rarely met. The solvents commonly used for the extraction of drugs include water, alcohol and their different dilutions.

(a) Water as a Solvent

Water is used as a solvent for the extraction of many types of active constituents such as proteins, gums, colouring agents, anthraquinone derivatives, many alkaloidal salts, glycosides, sugars and tannins. It can also dissolve enzymes, organic salts and organic acids but it can not dissolve fatty substances like waxes, fats, fixed oils and alkaloids (as free base).

Advantages

Water as solvent has the following advantages that :

(i) It is very cheap
(ii) It is non-toxic
(iii) It is non-inflammable
(iv) It can dissolve a wide range of chemical substances.

Disadvantages

(i) Water is not selective, as it can dissolve a wide range of substances some of which are not only medicinally inactive but many a times create stability problems.
(ii) Water is a good media for the growth of bacteria and molds therefore all preparations made with water must be suitably preserved by adding sufficient quantity of alcohol, chloroform, glycerin or sugar.
(iii) Water leads to hydrolysis of many substances.
(iv) Liquid extracts prepared with water require more heat for their concentration as compared to the extracts prepared with other solvents.

(b) Alcohol as a Solvent

Alcohol or ethanol can dissolve a large number of chemical

substances such as alkaloids, alkaloidal salts, glycosides, tannins, anthraquinone derivatives, volatile oils and resins but substances like albumin, gums, waxes, fats, most fixed oils and sucrose are insoluble in alcohol. Generally dilute alcohols (hydroalcoholic solutions) are used for many extractions but in some cases stronger alcohol may be used to prevent the extraction of unwanted substances such as gums etc.

Advantages

Alcohol as a solvent has the following advantages that :

(i) It is miscible with water in all proportions. Various dilutions of alcohol are used for extraction purposes. A mixture of alcohol and water is known as hydroalcoholic solution.

(ii) It is non-toxic in the quantities present in medicinal substances.

(iii) Bacteria and molds cannot grow in solutions containing 20% or more of alcohol.

(iv) Less heat is required for the concentration of extracts prepared with alcohol as compared to that of prepared with water.

(v) It is neutral hence preparations made with it are compatible with other products.

(vi) It is reasonably selective, e.g. in a drug containing a number of chemical substances such as alkaloidal salts, glycosides, albumin and gum, water will dissolve all the substances whereas dilute alcohol will dissolve only the alkaloidal salts and glycosides.

Disadvantages

The main disadvantage of alcohol is that it is costly as compared to water.

The other solvents used for the extraction of drugs include ether (anaesthetic ether), solvent ether, chloroform, glycerin, light petroleum, acids such as acetic acid and tannic acid, and propylene glycol.

9.2 Extraction processes

Extraction of crude drugs can be done by various processes depending on the physical nature of the drug and chemical properties of the constituents present in it. Various methods used for the extraction of drugs include :

1. Infusion
2. Decoction
3. Digestion
4. Maceration
5. Percolation.

The processes like infusion, decoction and digestion are now obsolete hence are rarely used with few exceptions for extraction of drugs. Only the maceration and percolation processes are of particular importance and most pharmacopoeias refer to these processes for the extraction of crude drugs.

1. Infusion

This method is used for those drugs which are soft in nature so that water may penetrate easily to the tissues and the active constituents are water soluble. The simplest form of apparatus consists of a beaker or a teapot but special pots known as infusion pots are also available. The drug to be extracted is placed at the bottom of the pot, water added and the contents stirred occasionally. Otherwise the drug may be enclosed in a piece of muslin and suspended just below the level of the water. The drug is allowed to remain in contact with water for the required time, usually 15 minutes. After the specified time, the liquid is strained and dispensed. The marc is not pressed to avoid expression of colloidal cells into the preparation and the final volume of the preparation is not adjusted by adding more of vehicle otherwise dilution of active constituents will take place.

Infusions must be freshly prepared and consumed within 24 hours of its preparation. Examples of infusions are infusion of senna and infusion of quassia.

Concentrated infusions differ from fresh infusions in that the concentrated infusions are prepared by maceration or percolation process and alcohol is used either as a menstruum or as a preservative. An infusion containing 20-25% alcohol can be stored for sufficient long time. Examples of concentrated infusions are : concentrated compound infusion of chirata and concentrated compound infusion of gentian.

2. Decoction

Decoction is the process in which the water soluble and heat stable constituents of hard and woody crude drugs are extracted out. Water is used as menstruum and the drug cut in small pieces is actually boiled with the menstruum for the stated time, usually 10 to 15 minutes. After boiling, the liquid is cooled and filtered, more water is passed through the marc to produce the required volume. Adjustment to final volume is necessary to get a uniform product because different workers will use different types of vessels and different sources of heat resulting in varying losses of water by evaporation. A freshly prepared decoction should only be dispensed and the same must be consumed within 24 hours. At present no decoction is official in 1P or BP.

3. Digestion

This process is a modified form of maceration in which the extraction of drugs is carried out by applying gentle heat to the substances being extracted. This method is applicable only to those drugs where moderately elevated temperature is not objectionable and the solvent action of the menstruum is increased by gentle heat.

4. Maceration

(a) Simple maceration for organised drugs Organised drugs are those drugs which have a specific cell structure like roots, stems, leaves, flowers etc.

In this process the extraction of drugs is carried out by placing the solid drugs (in suitable state of subdivision, either crushed, cut small or moderately coarse powder. Fine powders are not used because there will be difficulty in subsequent filtration) in contact with whole of the menstruum in a closed vessel for 2-7 days with occasional stirring. The liquid is strained and marc pressed, adding the expressed liquid to the strained liquid. The combined liquids are clarified by decantation or filtration. Final volume is not adjusted.

Water or alcohol is used as menstruum and closed vessel is used to prevent evaporation of the menstruum. The drug menstruum ratio is normally 1 : 10. Sufficient time is allowed for the menstruum to penetrate the plant tissues and for the soluble constituents to diffuse out. Stirring is necessary to disperse the concentrated layer of the dissolved constituents around the solid particles. The extracted liquids may contain small particles of insoluble cell contents therefore filtration is necessary to remove these particles but filtration should not be done too soon after extraction, the liquid should be allowed to stand for some time to settle any colloidal material and then filtered otherwise the liquid will again become cloudy due to coagulation of colloidal particles even after filtration. Preparations made by this process include : oxymel of squill, tincture of squill, tincture of lemon, tincture of orange etc.

(b) Simple maceration for unorganised drugs Unorganised drugs are those drugs which have no cellular or tissue structure and are obtained from plants as their exudates e.g. gums, resins, gum resins and oleogum-resins.

In this process the extraction of drugs is carried out by placing a weighed amount of drug in contact with 4/5th of the menstruum in a closed vessel for 2-7 hours with occasional shaking. After the specified period the clear liquid is decanted or filtered, the marc is not pressed, volume is adjusted by passing more of (remaining 1/5th) menstruum through the marc.

In case of unorganised drugs, the marc left behind after the extraction of active constituents forms a compact mass and does not retain any appreciable amount of menstruum therefore pressing the gummy residue is neither practicable nor necessary. The adjustment to volume by washing the gummy residue with more of menstruum leads to uniform composition. Preparations made by this process include compound tincture of benzoin, tincture of tolu and tincture of myrrh.

(c) Multiple maceration Repeated maceration may be more effective than single maceration because an appreciable amount of active constituents may be left behind in the first pressing of the marc which may be extracted out in the next maceration. It is established that maximum extraction is obtained in multiple maceration when the total quantity of menstruum to be used is divided in such a way that same quantity of menstruum is present during each maceration. However allowance must be made for the quantity of menstruum retained by the marc at the end of the process. Multiple maceration may be done by double or triple maceration processes.

(i) *Double maceration* During this process the maceration of the drug is carried out twice and the total volume of the menstruum to be used is divided in two parts in such a way that same quantity of menstruum is used for each maceration.

For first maceration the weighed amount of the drug is allowed to remain in contact with the specified amount of menstruum with occasional shaking for a definite time. After the time is over the liquid is strained and marc passed, combining the strained and expressed liquid. The 2nd part of menstruum is then added to the marc and allowed to stand for some time. The clear liquid is strained, marc pressed and liquids obtained from 1st and 2nd maceration are combined together, filtered and evaporated to get a product of required concentration. Concentrated compound infusion of gentian is prepared by double maceration process.

The equation for double maceration is :

$$\text{Volume of menstruum to be used for first maceration} = \frac{\text{Total volume of menstruum} - \text{Volume of mens-truum retained by the drug}}{2} + \text{Volume of men struum retained by the drug}$$

(ii) *Triple maceration* Triple maceration process is sometimes used where the marc cannot be pressed. As in double maceration, in the case of triple maceration, the menstruum is divided into three parts and maceration is done thrice. The equation for triple maceration is :

$$\text{Volume of menstruum to be used for first maceration} = \frac{\text{Total volume of menstruum} - \text{Volume of menstruum retained by the drug}}{3} + \text{Volume of menstruum retained by the drug}$$

$$\text{Volume f menstruum requird for second and third maceration} = \frac{\text{Total volume of menstruum} - \text{Volume of menstruum used for first maceration}}{2}$$

In this process a weighed amount of drug is allowed to remain in contact with the calculated amount of menstruum for a specified time with occasional shaking, the clear liquid is strained and reserved. Similarly second and third maceration is carried out by adding the calculated quantities of menstruum. The marc is pressed at the end of the third maceration and expressed liquid is mixed with the liquids obtained from the 2nd and 3rd maceration. The liquid obtained in the first maceration is quite concentrated as compared to the liquids obtained in 2nd and 3rd maceration hence the latter are combined and evaporated before mixing it with the first macerate. Before making up the final volume, alcohol 90% equal to 1/4th of the final volume of liquid to be prepared is added to prevent the growth of micro-organisms. Liquid extract of senna and concentrated infusion of quassia are prepared by triple maceration process.

5. *Percolation*

Percolation also known as simple percolation is another method of extraction of active constituents from the drugs used in the preparation of tinctures and liquid extracts. In this process the suitably comminuted drug is moistened with a sufficient quantity of menstruum, which is then packed in a percolator. The drug is allowed to remain in contact with the menstruum for 24 hours, then more of menstruum is added from the top and percolation is started. The required volume is collected, marc is pressed and expressed liquid is added to the percolate. The required volume is produced by adding more of menstruum and the mixed liquid is clarified by decantation or by filtration. Preparations made by percolation process are : tincture of belladonna, compound tincture of cardamom, strong tincture of ginger.

The entire percolation process is explained by dividing it into following stages :

(i) Size reduction or comminution of the drug The drug to be extracted is subjected to suitable degree of size reduction, usually from coarse powder to fine powder; to increase the surface area of the drug, for uniform packing of the percolator, to slow down the movement of the menstruum and to ensure complete exhaustion of the drug.

(ii) Imbibation During imbibation the powdered drug is moistened with a suitable amount of menstruum and allowed to stand for four hours in a well closed container. During this period the drug swells up and menstruum penetrates the cell walls. After the lapse of time, the moistened drug is passed through a coarse sieve to remove the lumps and to mix the dry powder, if any. This preliminary moistening of the drug is necessary because :

(a) The dried tissue swells when it come in contact with menstruum but if packed in the dry condition, subsequent swelling will reduce the porosity of the material and choke the percolator.

(b) The air present in the interstices is removed by menstruum, which will otherwise disturb the packing of the percolator due to which the menstruum will run mainly through the channels resulting in inefficient extraction.

(c) It does not allow the fine particles to be washed out of the percolator during percolation.

(iii) Packing After imbibation the moistened drug is evenly packed into a percolator. A percolator is a conical vessel having a lid at the top and is provided with a false bottom on which filter paper or cotton wool is placed to support the column of the drug and help in the escape of the percolate. The base of the percolator is fitted with a tap from which the percolate is collected. Two types of percolators are available (i) open percolator (ii) closed percolator. Open percolator is cheap and easy to handle. It is used when the menstruum is water or dilute alcohol. Closed percolator is used when the menstruum is volatile e.g. alcohol, ether etc. If the percolation is to be carried out at elevated temperatures then steam jacketed percolator may be used.

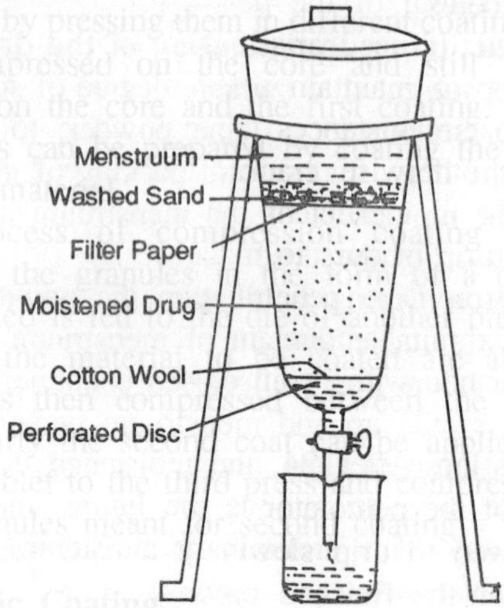

Fig. 9.1 Percolation

For packing, a piece of cotton wool, fibres of flax, hemp or any other suitable material; previously moistened with menstruum is placed on the false bottom of the percolator. A small amount (about 10%) of the moistened drug is introduced into the percolator and is pressed lightly with rod or any other suitable device, to give even compression. Similarly, more of moistened drug is introduced and pressed till whole of the drug is packed in the percolator. The packing should not be too tight, it will not allow the menstruum to pass freely which will lead to slow extraction rate. Similarly loose packing will allow the menstruum to pass through quickly resulting in incomplete contact with the drug, hence less dissolution of active constituents. Precaution should be taken that the drug should occupy about 2/3rd capacity of the percolator. After suitable packing of the drug into the percolator a piece of filter paper is placed over top of it on which small quantity of washed sand is placed to prevent disturbance of the packed material.

(iv) Maceration After packing the column, sufficient menstruum is added to saturate the material and top of the percolator is covered with a lid. When the liquid begins to drip from the bottom of the percolator, the tap fitted at its bottom is closed. If need arises then more of menstruum is added at the top to maintain a layer of menstruum over the drug. Under no circumstances the column should be allowed to become dry otherwise cracks will appear in the packed column resulting in inefficient percolation. The percolator is then set aside for 24 hours to macerate the drug. This period helps the menstruum to penetrate deep into the tissues and dissolve the maximum amount of active constituents and drug will be extracted with comparatively small volume of menstruum.

(v) Percolation After 24 hours maceration of the drug, the lower tap of the percolator is opened and liquid collected therein is allowed to drip slowly at a controlled speed until 3/4th volume of the finished product is obtained. Sufficient menstruum is simultaneously added over the drug because at no time packed material should be allowed to become dry. To avoid adding the menstruum time and again, a bottle full of menstruum carrying the delivery tube to the percolator may be fitted in the inverted position which will supply the menstruum continuously over the top of the percolator. After collecting 3/4th volume, the percolate is tested for complete exhaustion of the drug by various tests, the marc is then pressed and expressed liquid is added to the already collected percolate which should be about 80-90% of the final volume. More of menstruum is added to produce the required volume. The liquid is then allowed to stand to settle the suspended particles, decanted or clarified by filtration.

Tests to check complete exhaustion of the drug :

(i) Take a few ml of the last percolate and evaporate to dryness, if no residue remains this shows that the drug is completely exhausted.

(ii) Measure the specific gravity of last few ml of percolate if it is equal to the specific gravity of the menstruum, it shows exhaustion of the drug.

(iii) Specific tests may be performed on the percolate for the drugs containing alkaloids, glycosides, tannins, resins or bitter constituents.

9.3 Reserved Percolation

It is a percolation process in which first portion (about 3/4th of final product) of the percolate which contains the maximum amount of active constituents is reserved and subsequent percolation is completed as usual until the drug is exhausted but the last part, about 1/4th of final volume is collected separately. The second dilute part is then evaporated to get a syrupy consistency which is then mixed with the reserved portion of the percolate and the final volume is adjusted by adding more of menstruum.

Reserved percolation process is used for the preparation of liquid extracts as they are more concentrated preparations as compared to tinctures prepared by simple percolation process. Generally alcohol is used as menstruum for reserved percolation process and first portion of percolate which contains the bulk of dissolved active constituents is reserved and only the last portion which is dilute is subjected to evaporation, the concentrated product of which is mixed with the reserved part. Liquid extract of liquorice is prepared by this process.

Advantages

(i) The reserved part of percolate which contains the maximum amount of dissolved principles is not subjected to heat treatment for evaporation, only the dilute portion of percolate is evaporated.

(ii) This process is economical as whole of the percolate is not evaporated.

9.4 Continuous Hot Percolation Process or Soxhlet Extraction

Continuous hot percolation process is used for those drugs where the penetration of the menstruum into the cellular tissues is very slow and the solute is not readily soluble into the solvent and the quantity of menstruum is very less. In such cases Soxhlet extractor is used where small volume of hot menstruum is passed over the drug time and again to dissolve out the active constituents until the drug is exhausted. This process is known as Soxhlation.

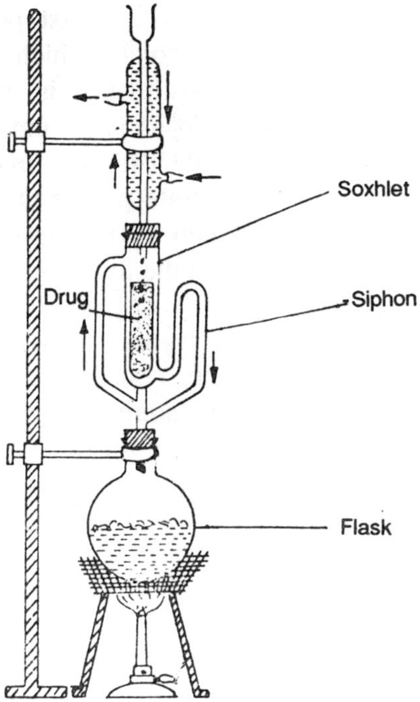

Fig. 9.2 Soxhlation

The Soxhlet apparatus required for the continuous hot percolation is made from a very high grade of glass and consists of three parts (a) a flask in which the menstruum is boiled (b) an extraction chamber in which drug is filled, is fitted with a side tube and a siphon (c) a condenser.

The drug to be extracted, in suitably comminuted form is usually packed in a 'thimble' made of filter paper which is then placed into the wider part of the extractor. 'Thimble' is used to prevent choking of the lower part of the extractor by drug particles. Menstruum is placed in the flask and boiled, the vapours are allowed to pass through the side tube to the condenser where they are condensed and fall on to the packed drug, through which it percolates and extract out the active constituents. As the volume of menstruum in the extractor increases, the level of the liquid in the siphon also increases till it reaches the maximum point from where it is siphoned out into the flask. On further heating, the menstruum vaporizes while the dissolved active constituents remain behind in the flask. The alternate filling and emptying of the body of the extractor goes on continuously till the drug is exhausted. Thus the same quantity of menstruum is made to percolate repeatedly, about 14 to 15 times through the drug and the active constituents are collected in the flask.

This process is not suitable for the drugs containing thermolabile active constituents.

9.5 Factors Affecting Selection of an Extraction Process

1. Nature of the Drug

The selection of an extraction process mainly depends on the physical nature of the drug. Hard and woody drugs are extracted by percolation process whereas soft drugs are extracted by maceration which is also suitable for the extraction of unorganised drugs. Percolation is not suitable for such drugs which may block the percolator.

2. Cost of the Drug

Costly drugs are extracted by percolation whereas cheaper drugs may be extracted by maceration. Cost involved in comminuting the drug should also be taken into consideration.

3. Stability of Drug

Continuous hot extraction process should not be used for those drugs the active constituents of which are thermolabile.

4. Therapeutic Value of the Drug

The drugs containing flavouring agents or bitters etc. which does not have much therapeutic value may be extracted by maceration but if the drug has considerable therapeutic value then percolation process should be used.

5. Nature of Solvent

If the solvent is water, maceration is generally adopted but if the solvent is volatile then percolation process should be used.

6. Concentration of the Product

Dilute preparations such as tinctures may be prepared by maceration or percolation but concentrated preparactions such as liquid extracts or dry extracts should be prepared by percolation or reserved percolation process.

9.6 Ayurvedic Dosage Forms

Like other systems of medicine Ayurvedic system also has different dosage forms like Arka, Kvatha, Churna, Bhasma etc. etc. The basic principles envolved in the preparation of these dosage forms are almost similar to those of allopathic processes like distillation, decoction, powders, calcination etc. etc. but their technique of preparation is litte-bit different from allopathic drugs. Various Ayurvedic dosage forms are described as follows :

1. Arka	Distillate
2. Kvatha	Decoction
3. Avaleha	Linctus
4. Asava Arista	Fermented preparations
5. Ghrita and Taila	Medicated ghee and oil
6. Varti/Anjana	Eye preparations
7. Churna	Fine powders
8. Pisti	Very fine powders
9. Bhasma	Calcinated residue
10. Vati/Gutika	Tablets and pills

1. Arka (Distillate)

It is prepared by distillation method and is used for fresh and soft drugs specially the flowers, the constituents of which get destroyed by boiling.

The drug to be extracted is thoroughly washed and wrapped in a muslin cloth. This cloth bag is kept in the water required for distillation (generally 8 times water is used for distillation). The apparatus is heated. When the distillation starts first few drops are not collected which may contain some impurities present in condenser or some unwanted volatile materials, then the vapours are condensed and collected in a receiver. When half part is collected then the distillation is stopped.

Dry and hard drugs are powdered and allowed to macerate. The macerated drug is put in the apparatus and water needed for distillation is added (here 10 times water is used). The distillate is collocated in a receiver.

In Ayuravedic system a vessel made up of copper or brass which has been tinned from inside is preferred. Examples of arka include : rose, kevra, fennel, sandal, peppermint etc. These can be used by incorporating in other form of drugs.

2. Kvatha (Decoction, Karra, Joshanda)

It is a liquid preparation which is prepared by decoction. This method is used for drugs which are free from volatile constituents. The drug is actually boiled in a vessel for 15-30 minutes, during boiling the contents are stirred. Then it is allowed to cool and filtered by passing through a muslin cloth.

The hard and woody drugs are comminuted to a coarse powder and macerated for 12 hours and then decoction is prepared. Kvathas are used for oral administration, fomentation action and for cleaning the wounds.

3. Avaleha (Linctus)

These are the semisolid or solid preparations prepared by evaporating the kvath. The kvath is evaporated to a semisolid consistency and then medicine is incorporated or it is further evaporated to get a solid product but care must be taken that the material does not stick to the evaporating pan. Avaleha may also be prepared by adding the medicine to simple syrup which is then evaporated to get a product of desired consistency.

For use the avaleha is eigher licked or placed over the tongue from where it is dissolved slowly in the mouth. Best example is Chyavanprash.

4. *Asava Arista (Fermented preparations)*

These are the liquid preparations which are prepared by fermentation process. Some of them are prepared without heat (asava) while others are prepared with heat (arista). Some preparations are sweet in taste while others are sour in taste e.g. vinegar.

For their preparation kvath, gur and honey are used. For imparting flavour to the preparation volatile substances or flavouring agents may be incorporated. The container in which these preparations are prepared should be made of wood. It is placed at a suitable place and a particular temperature is maintained throughout the fermentation period. It takes about one month for its preparation. After fermentation the material is filtered and stored in suitable cntainers.

These preparations are used to expel air through the anus, to increase flow of urine, to improve digestion and to make the body active. They are generally taken by mixing with an equal amount of water.

5. *Ghrita and Taila (Medicated ghee and oil)*

These are the liquid or semisolid dosage form of medicament which are meant for internal and external use. Medicated ghee is generally given internally as a general tonic and to remove constipation. The oils are applied externally for their antiseptic and fomentation action. They are extensively used for massage to a particular part or whole of the body.

6. *Varti/Anjana (Eye preparations)*

These are the solid dosage form of medicament which are meant for application to the eyes. Netar varti (meant for eyes) is an elongated solid preparation which is rubbed on a hard surface or stone with the help of a few drops of water and the contents are instilled into the eyes.

Anjana is a very fine powder meant for introduction into the eyes with the help of a glass stick. These preparations must be passed through a very fine sieve to remove gritty particles which otherwise may lead to irritation and discomfort to the eyes.

Some of the varties which are elongated in shape are meant for introduction into the rectum for expulsion of gases from stomach and to remove constipation. They can also be used for systemic or sedative action and in haemorrhoids.

7. Churna (Powders)

These are solid dosage form of medicament meant for internal use. These may be simple or compound. Simple churan contain only one medicament whereas compound churan contains two or more than two medicaments.

The dose is 2-3 gm which may be increased or decreased according to age and severity of disease. It is administered with water, milk, fruit juices or any other suitable liquid depending on the nature of disease. It may be given by mixing with gur or honey in equal quantity, with sugar twice the quantity and with milk four times the quantities as that of drug.

Precautions :

1. Thoroughly cleaned and dried drugs should be used for the preparation of churans.
2. They should be finely sifted.
3. Each substance should be powdered separately and then mixed.
4. Pestle and mortar used for reducing the particle size and mixing the substances should be clean and dry.
5. They must be stored in a dry container.
6. They should not be prepared in rainy season.
7. They should dissolve in the stomach contents.

8. Pisti (Very fine powder)

It is solid dosage form of medicament meant for internal use. It is prepared from very costly materials like diamond, pearls, monga, jaharmohra etc. These materials are thoroughly cleaned to remove sticking substances like dust etc. then they are reduced to a very fine powder using prolonged grinding which is then passed through a very fine sieve to remove gritty particles.

9. Bhasma (Calcinated residue)

It is solid dosage form of medicament meant for internal use. Generally pearls, iron, gold, silver, lead, tin, zinc, black mica etc are used for their preparation. The material is thoroughly cleaned and reduced to a coarse powder. The powdered material is mixed with a suitable liquid and kneaded to get a wet mass. This wet mass is rolled on a hard surface to get a pencil which is then divided into a number of pieces. Each piece is pressed in-between palms of hands to get large size tablets (slugs) These tablets are dried in sun light or in an oven. The dried tablets are put in earthen pots (kasore), two pots are used at a time, the mouths of which are combined together and the joint is sealed by surrounding it with cloth dipped in mud slurry and dried in the sun. Then these earthen pots are kept in the heap of cow dung cakes which are burnt afterwards. The material is allowed to heat in the burning fire for 12 hours which is then allowed to cool slowly while still in the fire. When the pots have cooled down they are removed from there and contents are taken out which are then ground by means of a machine, generally ball mill is used for this purpose.

10. Vati/Gutika (Tablets and pills)

These are solid dosage form of medicament(s) meant for oral administration prepared by hand or machine. The materials are mixed together and a suitable liquid is incorporated to make the mass wet. This wet mass is kneaded in-between the fingers so as to get a uniform mass. The mass so prepared is rolled on a hard surface so as to make a pencil which is then divided into desired number of pieces and each piece is rounded by fingers.

Precautions :

1. If the quantity of drugs is small the diluent may be added to increase the bulk. For potent drugs lactose may be used as diluent.
2. The material should be finely powdered.
3. Only soluble substances should be used which can dissolve in stomach.
4. Size should be within limits.
5. If pill breaks then a binding agent like gum acacia may be added.
6. To prevent sticking with each other cinnamon or glycyrrhiza powder should be sprinkled over the pills.
7. It should not be too soft or too hard.
8. Sugar coating should be done for volatile and bitter drugs.

Some of the commonly used Ayurvedic and Unani medicinal drugs/preparations include :

- Amla (Emblica officinalis)
- Banafsha (Viola odorata)
- Chyavanprash
- Guggal (Commiphora mukul)
- Haldi (Curcuma longa)
- Isphagula husk (Plantago ovata)
- Joshanda
- Khamira
- Lahsun (Allium sativum)
- Liv-52
- Mulethi (Glycyrrhiza glabra)
- Swarna bhasma (Calcinated gold)

10

Heat Processes

Heat, temperature and heat transfer are the three terms which are commonly used in pharmaceutical applications and must be defined in relation to each other. Heat is that form of energy which is transferred from one object to another when there is a difference in temperature between the two objects. Temperature is the degree of hotness or coldness of an object. When an object is heated, its temperature increases but when the object is cooled, its temperature decreases. Heat transfer refers to the actual flow of heat energy between the two objects. Heat energy flows from a system at higher temperature to a system at lower temperature.

Most of the pharmaceutical processes such as distillation, evaporation, drying, sterilization, extraction of volatile oils from crude drugs etc. require the application of heat. Heat is also required in the production of almost all types of formulations such as tablets, effervescent granules, syrups, glycerites, solutions, injections, ointments and suppositories at one stage or the other.

Heat is produced either by burning of solids such as coal; liquids such as petroleum products or gases like natural gas. Electricity is another major source of heat in which an electric current is passed through conductors with high resistances. Heating with electricity has gained wide importance over the conventional methods of heating which are relatively costlier. Other advantages of electrical heating include cleanliness of operation, easy handling, rapid response, uniform temperature control, ease in getting high temperatures, ready availability, ease of operation at any place and safety of operation.

Heating may either be done directly i.e. by keeping the vessel containing the material to be heated in direct contact with the source of heat or indirectly i.e. by keeping the vessel containing the material to be heated in a medium or bath which is heated. Different types of baths include water bath, sand bath, oil bath, glycerin bath, acid bath and steam bath. Direct heating is useful when high temperatures upto 1500°C is required and the material to be heated is thermostable. Indirect heating is done when the material is to be heated at particular temperature which can be thermostatically controlled.

10.1 Methods of Heat Transfer

Heat transfer from one system to another system can take place by three methods and all the three may occur simultaneously :

(i) Conduction
(ii) Convection
(iii) Radiation

(i) Conduction During conduction the transfer of heat from one part of a body to another part takes place by the transference of momentum of individual molecules, without any displacement of particles. The best example of transfer of heat by conduction is the heating up the whole length of rod when one end is heated and expanding of mercury of a thermometer when it is placed in a warm liquid.

(ii) Convection During convection the transfer of heat takes place from one point to another in a body of fluid by actual movement of particles i.e. a gas or a liquid circulates from one place to another as in mixing process. The best example of transfer of heat by convection is the heatlng of water in a glass beaker.

(iii) Radiation During radiation the transfer of heat energy from the source of heat to the object take place through space by means of electromagnetic waves, which travel in straight lines at the speed of light. The best example of transfer of heat by radiation is that we get heat from the sun by means of radiation and infra-red lamp transmits its heat by radiation.

10.2 Heat Processes

The important heat processes use in pharmaceutical manufacturing are discussed as under :

1. Evaporation
2. Sublimation
3. Exsiccation
4. Desiccation
5. Fusion
6. Calcination
7. Ignition
8. Distillation
9. Freeze drying

1. Evaporation

Theoretically, evaporation means the free escape of vapours from the surface of a liquid below its boiling point. It is a slow process and can take place even at room temperature. Since evaporation is too slow at room temperature, so the liquid is boiled from where the vapours escape in the form of bubbles from the bulk of the liquid.

Thus practically evaporation may be defined as the removal of liquid from a solution by boiling the solution in a suitable vessel from where the vapours are withdrawn and a concentrated liquid is left behind. Evaporation is maximum at the boiling point of the substance.

Evaporation differs from boiling that evaporation takes place at all temperatures whereas boiling takes place only at one temperature at a given pressure. Evaporation occurs only at the surface of the liquid whereas in the case of boiling, evaporation takes place from whole of the liquid. Boiling occurs when the vapour pressure of the liquid becomes equal to the atmospheric pressure. Evaporation differs from distillation that in evaporation the solvent which is generally water is not condensed and collected whereas in distillation the solvent vapours are condensed and are collected in a receiver.

10.3 Factors Affecting Evaporation

(i) Temperature The rate of evaporation is directly proportional to the temperature. Higher the temperature higher will be evaporation but evaporation is maximum at the boiling point of the liquid. Thermostable preparations can be evaporated at high temperatures but thermolabile preparations will have to be evaporated at low temperatures. Many substances like glycosides, alkaloids, hormones, enzymes and antibiotics may get decomposed even at temperatures below 100°C hence they should be evaporated at a careful temperature. Extremely heat sensitive substances may be evaporated under reduced pressure.

The time required for evaporation is very critical. Exposure to a high temperature for a short period of time may be less destructive than a lower temperature with exposure for a longer period. Therefore as far as possible evaporation should be carried out for short time at low temperature.

Some drugs decompose more readily in the presence of moisture, specially at a raised temperature. Similarly hydrolysis and many other degradation reactions take place in the presence of moisture. Therefore evaporation in some cases may be carried out at a low controlled temperature till a concentrated product is obtained and final drying, when little moisture remains, may be done at higher temperatures.

(ii) Surface area The rate of evaporation is directly proportional to the surface area of the vessel exposed to evaporation. Greater the surface exposed to evaporation higher will be the rate of evaporation.

(iii) Agitation During evaporation the upper layers of the liquid to be evaporated has a tendency to form a scum or layer which lowers the rate of evaporation. Therefore it becomes necessary to agitate or stir the solution under evaporation. This will also prevent the decomposition of the preparation at the bottom due to excessive heat and will also prevent the settling of the solids at the bottom of the container.

(iv) Atmospheric aqueous vapour pressure If the atmospheric aqueous vapour pressure or moisture contents in the air are high, the rate of evaporation will be slow but if it is less then evaporation will be fast. Therefore rate of evaporation can be increased by free circulation of warm air over the evaporating pan.

(v) Atmospheric pressure on the liquid under evaporation The rate of evaporation is inversely proportional to the atmospheric pressure on the surface of the liquid. If the atmospheric pressure on the liquid is reduced to half then the rate of evaporation will be doubled. Due to this reason in many cases the evaporation is done under reduced pressure i.e. by producing vacuum over the surface of the liquid.

(vi) Type of product required The selection of the method and apparatus to be used for evaporation depends upon the type of product required. Evaporating pans or stills may be used to produce liquid or dry products but film evaporators may be used to get liquid products.

(vii) Economic factors While selecting the method and apparatus employed for evaporation, due consideration must be given to economy of labour, fuel, floor area and materials. The recovery of solvents and the utilisation of "waste" heat are also important factors which contribute significantly in the reduction of overall costs.

10.4 Evaporators

Small Scale Methods

Small quantities of liquids may be evaporated in a porcelain or glass dish. Generally direct heating by bunsen burner or electric hot plate is used for evaporation but it should not be employed, as direct heating leads to decomposition of the substances towards the end of evaporation. A fixed maximum temperature can easily be attained by employing different types of baths as a source of indirect heating. A water bath is most suitable when the liquids are to be heated upto 100°C. They are simple and inexpensive and there is no risk of charring the materials. Sand bath or oil bath containing liquid paraffin or soft paraffin may be used when higher temperatures upto 300°C are required. Glycerin bath is used to attain a temperature upto 150°C. To prevent decomposition, whole of the liquid should not be evaporated to dryness. The last traces of solvent from the concentrated liquid may be removed under controlled temperatures. The evaporation of large quantities of liquids or solutions having costly solvents should be carried out by distillation under reduced pressure.

Large Scale Methods

(i) Evaporating pans On a manufacturing scale, liquid extracts containing water as a menstruum are evaporated in open pans called evaporating pans. They consist of hemispherical or shallow pans made of copper, stainless steel, aluminium, enamelled iron or other metal and surrounded by a steam jacket. Pans made from stainless steel and jacket from cast iron is most suitable. To prevent rusting of the later, the iron is enamelled on the inner surface. The hemispherical shape is most suitable because it affords the best surface/volume ratio for heating. These pans may be fixed or made to tilt to remove the product.

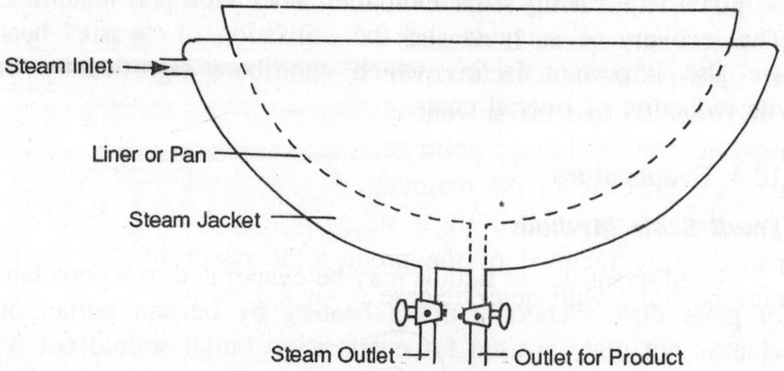

Fig. 10.1 Evaporating pan

For convenience in emptying the fixed pans, a tube passes from the lowest point of liner, through the jacket, which is fitted with a tap to withdraw the evaporated liquid from the pan, as and when desired.

Advantages

1. They are simple, easy and cheap to construct.
2. They are easy to use and clean.
3. Stirring of the evaporating liquids can be done easily.

Disadvantages

1. The whole of the liquid is heated all the time which may lead to decomposition of the components.
2. On the evaporating surface, scum is rapidly formed which decreases evaporation. Solids may be deposited at the bottom which makes the stirring necessary.
3. These pans can only be used for evaporating aqueous and thermostable liquid extracts. They cannot be used for evaporating extracts containing organic solvents like alcohol etc.
4. The room in which evaporating pans are used for evaporating the liquids, must be fitted with efficient exhaust fans otherwise the room will be filled with dense fog of condensed vapours and water will start falling from the roof and along the sides of the walls.

(ii) Evaporating stills Evaporating stills are quite similar to evaporating pans. It consists of a vessel made from copper or stainless steel, with a cover which is fitted with a water condenser so that the solvent is condensed and collected in a receiver. At the lowest point of the pan, a tube fitted with a tap is connected for the removal of the product from the pan. The pan is surrounded by a steam jacket. For cleaning the pan or easy removal of the product the cover of the vessel may be fitted with quick-release system of clamps.

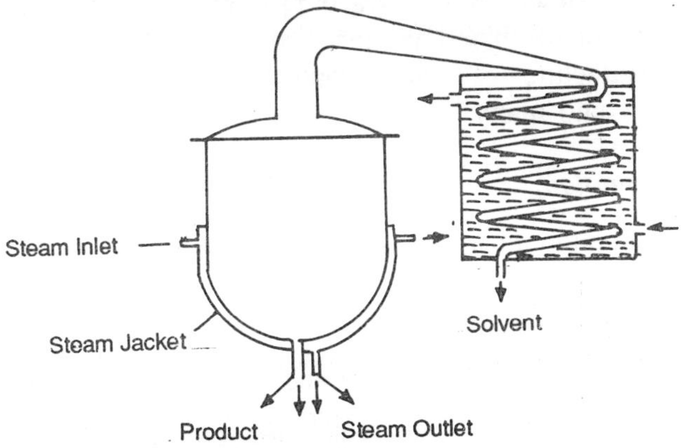

Fig. 10.2 Evaporating still

Advantages

1. They are very simple to construct and are quite easy to clean and maintain.
2. As the vapours are condensed, it increases the rate of evaporation.
3. A receiver and vacuum pump can be fitted to the apparatus by which evaporation under reduced pressure can be carried out and at low temperatures.
4. The still can be used for evaporating liquids containing aqueous and other organic solvents.
5. Since the cover can be removed easily therefore the still may be conveniently used for evaporating extracts to dryness.

Disadvantages

1. The whole of the liquid is to be heated all the time which may lead to deterioration of the product.
2. The heating surface is very limited.

This method of evaporation is widely used in pharmaceutical industries when small batches of liquids are to be evaporated.

Applications of Evaporation

Evaporation is one of the most important processes in the manufacture of pharmaceuticals. It is used in the preparation of liquid extracts, soft extracts and dry extracts and in the concentration of blood plasma and serum. It is also used in the manufacture of drugs containing antibiotics, enzymes, hormones and many other substances.

2. Sublimation

Sublimation is the process in which, on heating, a solid gets converted to vapours without intermediate formation of a liquid state and on condensation, the vapours get converted back to the solid state. The product so obtained is known as sublimate.

A solid sublimes only when the pressure on a solid is lower than the triple point, i.e. a solid is converted to vapours and on condensation a solid is obtained, this is called "true sublimation". But when pressure on a solid is higher than the triple point, liquid phase will be produced before conversion into vapours and then to solids, this is called "sublimation". The triple point mentioned here is the point, having a definite pressure and temperature, at which the solid, liquid and vapour phases of a chemical substance can co-exist indefinitely.

Method of Sublimation

No specific device or apparatus is required. On laboratory scale sublimation may be carried out by using a very simple apparatus consisting of a china dish, a perforated filter paper, a funnel and a plug of cotton wool. The material to be sublimed is put in the china dish which is covered with a perforated filter paper. A glass funnel, the open end of which is plugged with cotton wool, to prevent the escape of sublimed product; is placed in the inverted position over the filter paper. The china dish is heated over sand bath and vapours pass through the perforations of the filter paper which are collected on the inner surface of the glass funnel which is kept cool from outside by wrapping a wet filter paper or cotton wool. The vapours on cooling are condensed into a solid which is collected afterwards.

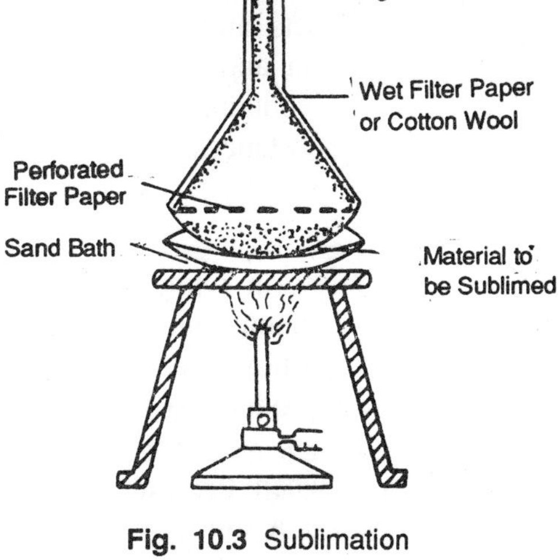

Fig. 10.3 Sublimation

In certain cases, to prevent the decomposition of substances due to high temperatures, sublimation can be done at low temperatures under reduced pressure.

Applications

1. The process of sublimation is used in the purification of many pharmaceutical substances such as iodine, camphor, mercuric chloride, mercurous chloride and sublimed sulphur.
2. It is also used in the manufacture of iodine, ammonium chloride and naphthalene.
3. This process is also employed to purify volatile solids contaminated with non-volatile impurities.

3. Exsiccation

Exsiccation is the process of removing the water of crystallization from the hydrated crystalline substances and making them anhydrous. The examples of exsiccated substances include exsiccated ferrous sulphate, exsiccated magnesium sulphate, exsiccated sodium sulphate, exsiccated sodium carbonate, exsiccated alum and anhydrous sodium arsenate.

In the laboratory, exsiccation may be carried out by taking a weighed amount of the substance in a tared dish which is heated on water bath, sand bath or in an oven, with continuous stirring until a constant weight is obtained or until the calculated loss in weight has taken place.

The temperature required to remove water of crystallization is very important. For example, copper sulphate, $CuSO_4 . 5H_2O$, when heated at about 30°C loses two molecules of water of crystallization, at 100°C it loses two more water molecules and the last water molecule is removed when it is heated at 200°C, thus forming $CuSO_4 . 3H_2O$, $CuSO_4.H_2O$ and $CuSO_4$ respectively. Similarly ferrous sulphate $FeSO_4.7H_2O$ when heated on water bath loses six molecules of water of crystallization but when further heated to remove last water molecule, decomposition takes place. Hence ferrous sulphate with one molecule of water of crystallization $FeSO_4.H_2O$ is called exsiccated ferrous sulphate.

Since the exsiccated salts are very hygroscopic, so must be stored in well closed containers.

Applications

1. Exsiccation is done to get an anhydrous product required in the formulation of certain medicaments.
2. It is also carried out to reduce the bulk and weight of certain drugs so that they can be easily administered.
3. Generally on exsiccation a fine powder of the substance is obtained.

4. Desiccation

Desiccation is the process of removing adhered moisture from liquid or solid substances. The term "desiccated" should be used for those substances from which water has been completely removed.

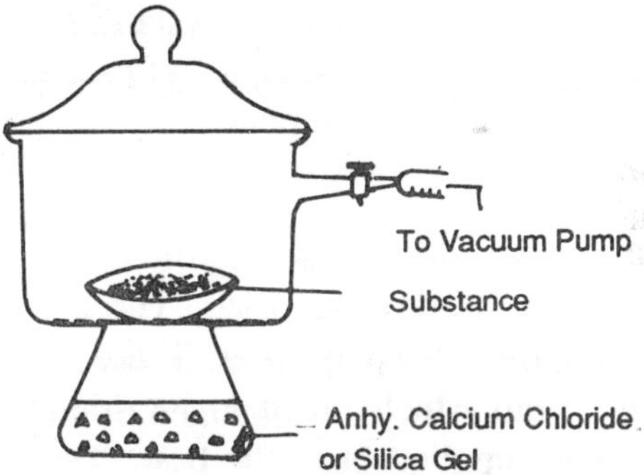

Fig. 10.4 Desiccation

On laboratory scale desiccation can be carried out in a desiccator which consists of a tightly closed glass vessel containing a drying agent at its bottom, which absorbs moisture from the substance being desiccated. The commonly used drying agents include concentrated sulphuric acid, phosphorous pentoxide, exsiccated calcium chloride and silica gel. The drug to be dried is taken in a dish which is placed inside the desiccator above the surface of drying agent. For continuous operation the desiccator may sometimes be connected to a vacuum pump.

The substances which are very sensitive to moisture are formulated as tablets or capsules which are further protected by enclosing them in sealed vials, on the bottom of which a small cloth bag containing silica gel is placed which acts as a desiccant. The last traces of moisture from some of the organic solvents is removed by passing through a column of alumina or silica gel.

Applications

1. Desiccation helps in preserving the vegetable and animal drugs which get destroyed in the presence of moisture.
2. Comminution of drugs is difficult if they are wet but if they are dry, can be easily powdered.
3. Desiccation reduces the bulk and weight of the substances due to loss of adhering moisture in them therefore they become easy to handle.
4. Stability of certain drugs is also increased.

Spray Drying

Spray drying is one of the methods of desiccation by which solutions or slurries are dried. The apparatus used for this purpose is known as spray drier. These driers consist of a hot air chamber into which liquid to be dried is fed from the top and hot air is supplied from the base. The spraying of the liquid is done either by pressure jets or by high speed rotors, of which latter are better because pressure jets tend to get choked. By the high current of hot air the liquid is sprayed in the form of a mist, the droplets of which are readily evaporated and the dried particles fall to the bottom of the chamber from where they are collected. The exhausted air leaves the chamber through the air outlet.

Different types of spray driers are available with various modifications. In some forms of spray driers the liquid to be dried and hot air enters from the top of the chamber and in others from the bottom. Still in other types liquid is fed from the top and hot air from the bottom.

Applications

1. These driers are very useful because the drying is very rapid as large surface of liquid is exposed to hot air and temperature required for drying is also low. Therefore heat sensitive products can be dried conveniently.
2. Spray drying is used for drying blood plasma, milk and enzyme preparations such as pancreatin and pepsin.
3. Spray driers can be designed for drying under sterile conditions.
4. Encapsulation of solid and liquid particles can be done by spray drying.

5. *Fusion*

Fusion is the process by which the solids gets converted into liquids without adding any solvent. It may also be defined as the process of heating the solids until they melt.

Fusion is done to purify certain solid and semisolid substances e.g. bees wax, hard paraffin, soft paraffin and wool fat are heated to melt and filtered while hot, to remove the dissolved impurities. On cooling, a product free from dissolved impurities is obtained. This method is also applied for the preparation of ointments when they also contain solids and semisolids in the formulation. All the substances are melted and then cooled slowly with continuous stirring until a uniform product is obtained. To avoid overheating substances with higher melting points are melted first to which substances with lower melting points are added.

6. *Calcination*

Calcination is the process in which the inorganic substances are strongly heated so as to remove their volatile contents and a fixed residue is obtained. On laboratory scale calcination is done in silica or platinum crucibles whereas in industries metallic vessels are used.

Calcination is used in the preparation of certain inorganic substances such as calcium oxide, light magnesium oxide, heavy magnesium oxide, zinc oxide and red mercuric oxide.

These substances are prepared by heating their respective carbonates. This method is also used in gravimetric analysis of certain pharmaceutical preparations.

7. *Ignition*

Ignition or incineration is the process by which an organic substance is strongly heated until whole of carbonaceous matter burns and an inorganic residue know as ash is left behind. On laboratory scale ignition is carried out in silica or platinum crucibles.

This process is mainly used for the standardization of organic substances and crude drugs by means of gravimetric analysis.

11
Distillation

Distillation is the process of separating the constituents of a liquid by vaporizing the liquid and passing the vapours through a cold surface thereby converting the vapours again to a liquid. Hence it involves a change of state from liquid to vapour and again to liquid. The vessel or the container in which the liquid is heated is known as still which is connected to an apparatus through which cold water is circulated to afford condensation called condenser. The vessel in which the condensed liquid is collected is known as receiver and the liquid so received is called distillate. On laboratory scale the distillation apparatus i.e. still, condenser and receiver is generally made of glass but it may also be made from a metal best suited to the process.

11.1 Difference Between Distillation and Evaporation

Distillation differs from evaporation that :

(i) In distillation the liquid from which the vapour arises is heated to boiling point and maintained at this temperature throughout the process and vapour formation occurs throughout the liquid. Whereas in evaporation the liquid is maintained below its boiling point and the vapour formation occurs only at the surface of the liquid.

(ii) In distillation the vapours are passed through a condenser to re-obtain the liquid. Whereas in evaporation the vapours are not condensed to re-obtain the liquid.

Condensers

The selection of a suitable condenser is necessary for the success of many distillation processes. An ideal condenser should have the following characteristics :

(i) The construction of the condenser should be such that it can be easily cleaned so as to remove even traces of previous product.

(ii) The broken parts may be easily replaced so that the cost of a new condenser is saved.

(iii) It should provide the maximum cooling surface because the rate of condensation is directly proportional to the cooling area.

(iv) Condensing surface should be good conductor of heat therefore where practicable metal condensers are preferred than glass condensers.

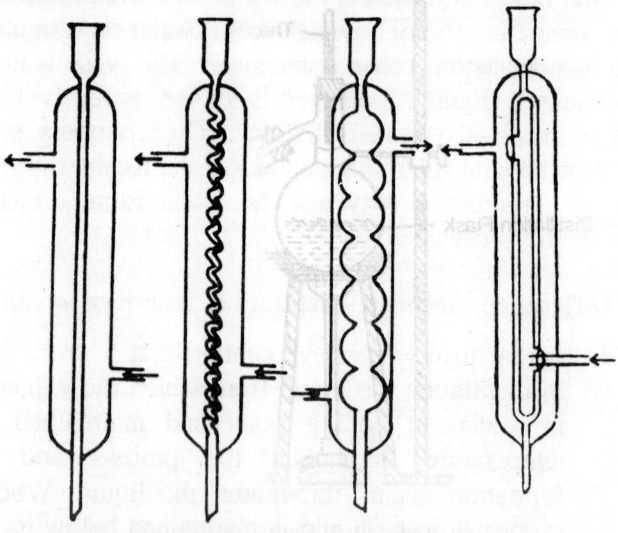

Fig. 11.1 Condensers : (1) Liebig condenser (2) Spiral condenser (3) Bulb condenser (4) Double surface condenser

(v) The water used for cooling the surface must leave the condenser quickly so, as to provide space for fresh water to get in and provide cold surface. The cooling water must flow in the opposite direction to that of vapours to be condensed so that the condensed liquid should leave the condenser in as cool a condition as possible.

The various types of condensers used for distillation include Leibig condensers, spiral condensers, bulb condensers, double surface condensers and multitubular condensers. Diagrammatically these condensers are shown in Fig 11.1

11.2 Types of Distillation

Different types of distillation are :

(i) Simple distillation
(ii) Fractional distillation
(iii) Steam distillation
(iv) Distillation under reduced pressure (Vacuum distillation)
(v) Destructive distillation.

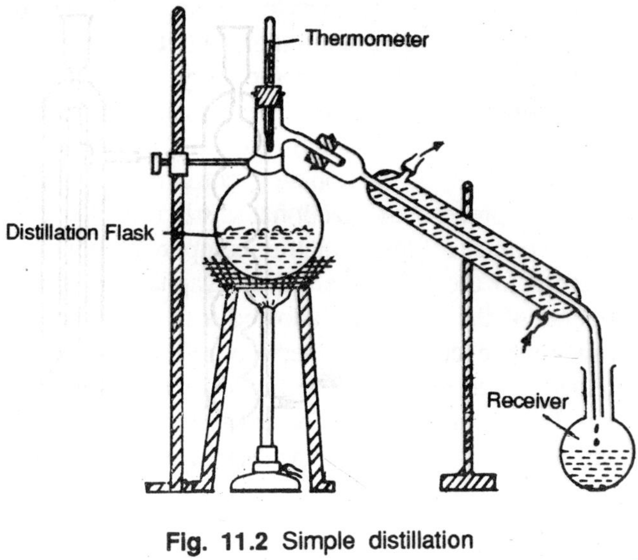

Fig. 11.2 Simple distillation

(i) Simple distillation Simple distillation is the process of converting a liquid into its vapours which are passed through a cooling surface to condense the vapours. The condensed vapours are reformed into a liquid which is collected in a receiver. The apparatus generally used for simple distillation consists of still, the condenser and the receiver. Depending on the suitability, the apparatus may consist of glass or a metal.

Applications

Simple distillation is mainly used for the purification of organic liquids and for the separation of liquids from non-volatile solids e.g. recovery of alcohol in the preparation of dry extracts. This process is also used in the preparation of ether, amyl nitrate and spirit of nitrous ether.

Distilled water is an important product which is prepared by simple distillation process.

(ii) Fractional distillation Fractional distillation process is used to separate miscible volatile liquids having different boiling points e.g. a mixture of alcohol and water. Alcohol is more volatile than water, therefore, will evaporate at a faster rate than water. It is quite easy to separate a liquid from non-volatile solids by simple distillation but it is very difficult to separate two volatile liquids completely from each other by simple distillation. Such type of miscible liquids can be separated by using fractionating columns in between the still and the condenser. A fractionating column is a device which increases the process of fractional distillation by condensing most of vapours of less volatile component of the mixture and return it to the still, whereas the vapours of more volatile components of the liquid are allowed to pass to the condenser. The vapours are condensed there to reform the liquid which is collected in the receiver. The liquid collected in the receiver may not be a pure liquid. Therefore repeated distillation of the distillates may have to be carried out to get a pure product.

Applications

Fractional distillation process is used in the separation of two immiscible liquids having different boiling points. It is also used in the manufacture of alcohol by means of a special form of still known as Coffey's still.

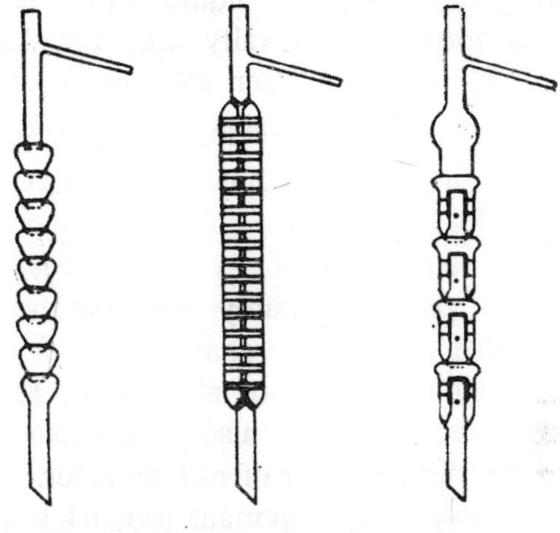

Fig. 11.3(a) Fractionating columns

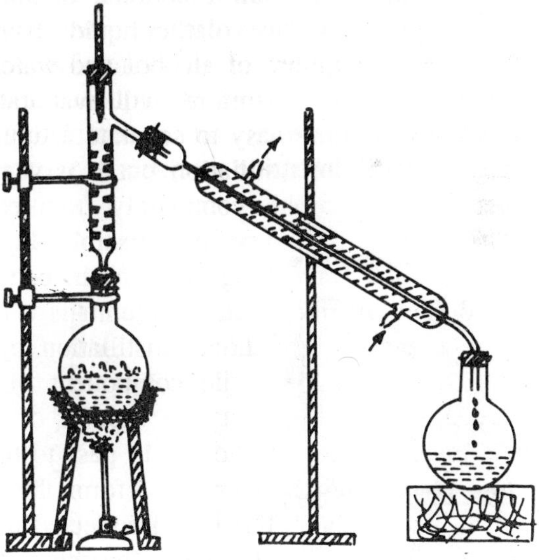

Fig. 11.3(b) Fractional distillation

(iii) Steam distillation Steam distillation is used for the distillation of two immiscible liquids one of which is water. An immiscible liquid and water independently boils at high temperature but when steam is passed through a mixture of these liquids, it boils at a much lower temperature than the boiling point of pure water. Thus turpentine which has a boiling point of about 160°C, when mixed with water can be distilled at about 95.6°C if a current of steam is passed through it.

On laboratory scale the distillation apparatus consists of steam generator fitted with a rubber bung having two holes. Through one hole a long safety tube is passed which permits the expulsion of some water if excessive pressure is generated inside the steam generator. Escape of steam from the safety tube indicates that the steam can is almost dry. Through the other hole a bent tube is passed which carries the steam to the flask containing the liquids (volatile liquid and small quantity of water) to be distilled. This tube must dip almost to the bottom of the flask. The steam can and flask containing the liquids are heated simultaneously so that a rapid current of steam passes through the boiling mixture in the flask. The vapours are allowed to pass through the condenser and condensed liquids are collected in Florentine receiver. The distillate which forms two layers, one aqueous and other non-aqueous are separated from each other as completely as possible. For this purpose either Florentine receivers or separating funnels are used.

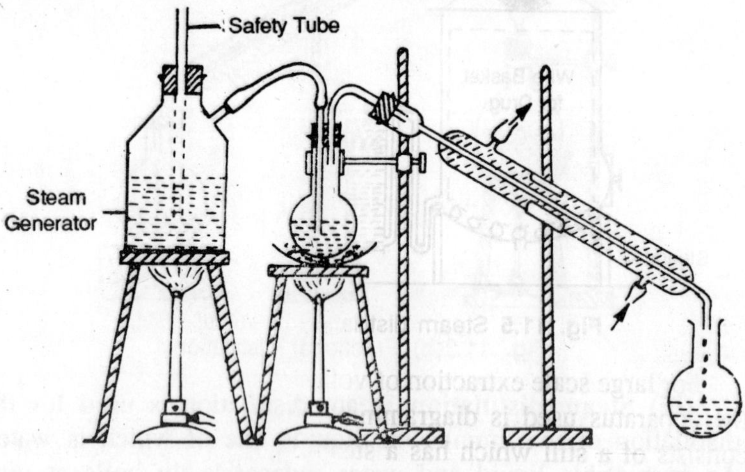

Fig. 11.4 Steam distillation

Florentine receiver is a specially designed receiver meant for collecting the oil and water in the same receiver. They are of two types, one type is used for separating oils lighter than water and the other one is used for separating oils heavier than water. The former is fitted with a siphon at the bottom and a tap at the top. As the distillate collects in the receiver and when it is filled, the siphon starts working by which only the water leaves the receiver and the oil which is collected at the top is removed by opening the tap fitted over there. The later type of receiver is fitted with a tap at the bottom as well as at the top. The oil which is heavier than water is collected from the lower tap and water is collected from the tap fitted near the top.

Steam distillation is used for the extraction of most of volatile oils such as clove oil, anise oil and eucalyptus oil etc. The extraction is done on the same principle that when steam is passed through a mixture of immiscible liquids, the mixture boils below the normal boiling point of either component.

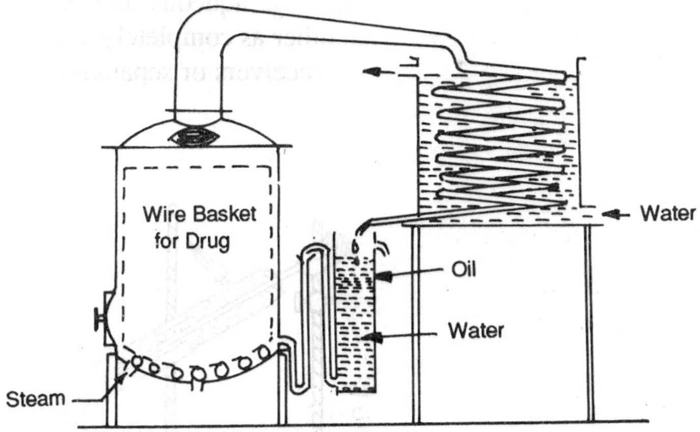

Fig. 11.5 Steam distillation of volatile oils

For large scale extraction of volatile oils by steam distillation the apparatus used is diagrammatically shown in Fig. 11.5. It consists of a still which has a steam jacket. The drug, suitably comminuted is placed in the wire basket which is kept in the still through the manholes provided at the top and side. The steam is introduced to the jacket of the still and water present there is made to boil. At this point steam is introduced into the still itself through the free-steam pipe. The oil-vapours and steam are passed through the condenser where they are converted into liquids which are collected in the Florentine receiver from where oil and water are mechanically separated and water is returned to the still.

Applications

Steam distillation is used for the distillation of water immiscible liquids of high boiling points e.g. turpentine and aniline. It is also used for the extraction of volatile oils from their crude drugs e.g. clove, anise and eucalyptus etc. Steam distillation is also useful for the purification of volatile substances.

(iv) Distillation under reduced pressure (Vacuum distillation) Distillation under reduced pressure or vacuum distillation works on the principle that a liquid boils when its vapour pressure is equal to the atmospheric pressure or external pressure. From this it is clear that the liquids which are decomposed at their boiling point under atmospheric pressure can be distilled at a much lower temperature than its boiling point if the pressure is reduced on the surface of the liquid. Boiling under reduced pressure will also increase the rate of distillation.

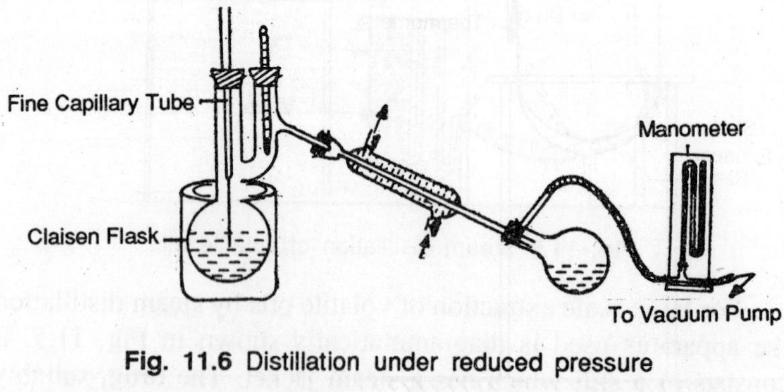

Fig. 11.6 Distillation under reduced pressure

Distillation under reduced pressure is carried out in a specially designed flask known as Claisen flask. This flask has two necks. Through one neck a thermometer is inserted and is attached to the condenser. Through the other neck a very fine capillary is introduced which completely dips in the boiling liquid. During distillation under reduced pressure, bumping occurs very readily which can be easily prevented by introducing a stream of air bubbles into the liquid through the capillary. The side tube of the receiver is connected to a vacuum pump to provide suitable vaccum. During vacuum distillation a small pressure gauge (manometer) should be inserted in between the receiver and the vacuum pump. For distillation, heating of the flask should not be started until the required vacuum has been attained above the surface of the liquid otherwise frothing of the hot liquid will result in the receiver. Preferably heating of the flask should be done on water bath or oil bath maintained at about 20°C higher than the boiling point of the liquid. During vacuum distillation thin walled glass apparatus like ordinary flat bottomed flasks and conical flasks should never be used otherwise collapsing of such apparatus may result.

Vacuum Stills

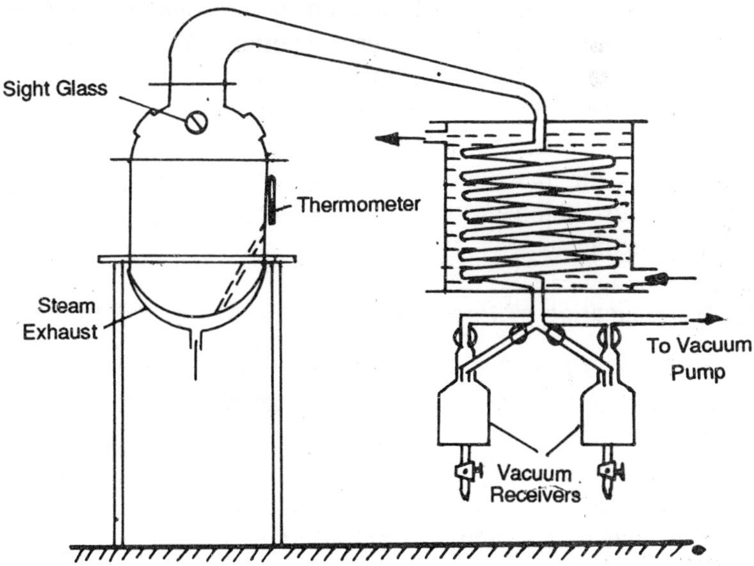

Fig. 11.7 Vacuum still

These are used for large scale distillation under reduced pressure. They are employed for those substances which have high boiling point at atmospheric pressure and get destroyed at high temperatures.

Vacuum stills consist of steam-jacketed stills made of copper, stainless steel or glass and are provided with a sight glass "observation window" to help the operator to see the progress of distillation. A tap is provided near the hood of the still for filling the still. The reduction in pressure is effected by means of mechanical air pumps driven by electricity. For easy collection and removal of distillate without stopping the distillation, two or three receivers are used which are fitted with suitable arrangement of cocks. These stills vary in design and are specially manufactured for the specified job. All the valves and cocks fitted in the vacuum stills should be of very high quality.

Applications

This process is used for the distillation of thermolabile substances and is also commonly used for the concentration and drying of extracts which get destroyed at high temperatures.

(v) Destructive distillation During this process the decomposition of usually natural products is carried out by heat and the volatile products of decomposition are condensed and collected. Though it is not a pharmaceutical process but is used in the destructive distillation of wood and coal to produce tars which are ultimately used in the preparation of certain medicines.

11.3 Preparation of Purified Water and Water for Injection

In majority of the liquid formulations water is used as vehicle. It is also used as a solvent for a number of drugs. Water is used because it is tasteless, free from irritating qualities and does not possess any pharmacological actions. Ordinary drinking water usually contains traces of dissolved salts of calcium and magnesium and traces of dissolved gases which include carbon dioxide and ammonia. Water obtained from different sources differ in these dissolved impurities and when combined with drugs leads to certain decomposition reactions. Therefore tap water is unsuitable for mal.ing pharmaceutical preparations hence drinking water must be purified before using in the pharmaceuticals and distilled water is therefore indicated for this purpose. Such water must comply with limit tests for chlorides, sulphates, iron, copper, lead, oxidizable matter, total solids and ammonia. Distilled water may be prepared from drinking water by distillation, by the use of ion-exchange resins or by reverse osmosis.

The use of purified water for pharmaceutical purposes is so great that it becomes necessary to prepare this water by a continuous process. A typical form of distillation unit for the continuous preparation of purified water is shown in Fig. 11.8. This type of still is known as Stoke's still.

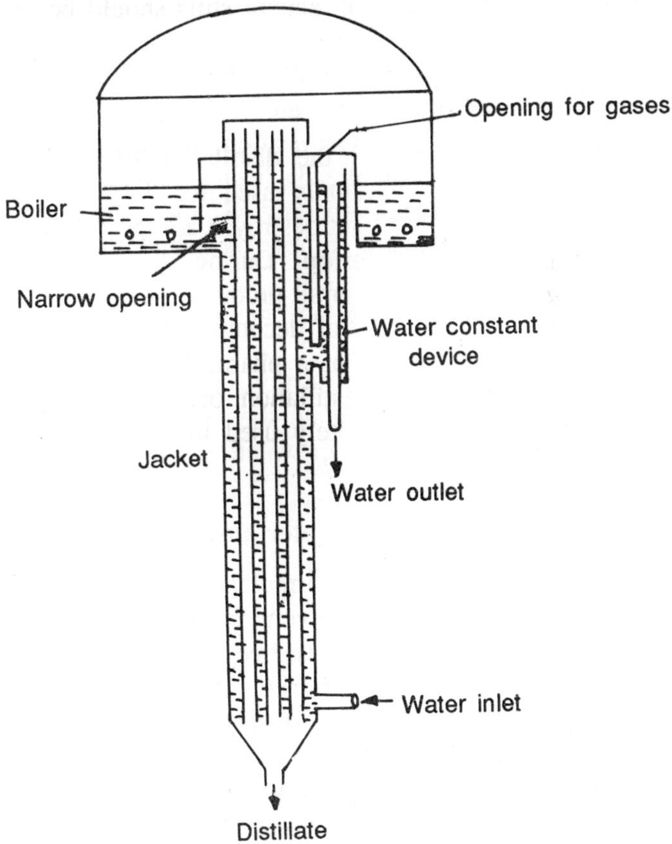

Fig. 11.8 Stokes still

The boiler of the still may consist of cast iron but the baffles and condenser tubes which come in contact with the product should be made from stainless steel or enamelled metal. The cold water from the water tap enters the still through an opening A, which rises in the Jacket B fitted with a constant-level device C, the excess of water over flows through the outlet D. The constant level device is attached to the boiler so as to prevent excessive concentration of salts, the volatile constituents of which may contaminate the product. Since some dissolved solids will be deposited along the sides of the boiler and on heating coils therefore it becomes necessary to remove such deposited solids from there, periodically, the frequency of which depends on the hardness of the feed water. A Portion of hot water at 90 to 95°C enters into the boiler E through an opening F—the level of water is maintained in the boiler upto overflow level. The water is boiled in the boiler E by means of heating coils. On heating, the dissolved gases, major portion of which has already been removed are allowed to escape through a small opening G and only the steam escapes into the condensing tubes, the condensed water is collected at H.

Since the dissolved gases are more volatile than water, they escape in the first portion of the distillate therefore must be rejected. Similarly the last portion of the distillate should also be rejected as it may contain the volatile portion of the dissolved solid substances in tap water.

Water for Injection

Water for injection is prepared by fitting baffles (an efficient device for preventing the entrainment of liquid droplets containing pyrogens) in the path of vapours between the boiler and the condenser. For preparing water for injection distillation still made from a neutral glass or stainless steel fitted with baffles is preferred. The distillate collected is immediately sterilized by heating in an autoclave or by filtration without the addition of a bactericide.

When water for injection free from carbon dioxide is required, the distillate should be boiled for 10 minutes with minimum exposure to air which can be achieved by covering the mouth of the flask with a small beaker in the inverted position. The boiled water is then cooled and distributed in the final containers which should be immediately sterilized by heating in an autoclave.

Ion exchange processes are also used for the preparation of purified water which can be used for all pharmaceutical purposes except in those preparations where water for injection is required. This is due to the reason that during ion exchange processes the pyrogens are not effectively removed.

12
Drying Processes

Drying is an important process in almost all the pharmaceutical industries. There is hardly any pharmaceutical plant engaged in the manufacture of tablets or capsules that does not use dryers. Drying is commonly the last stage of the process before packaging and has a considerable effect on the properties of the product which may prevent the deterioration, produce a readily soluble or free flowing product.

Drying is defined as a process in which the liquid is removed from a material by the application of heat and is accomplished by the transfer of a liquid from a surface into an unsaturated vapour phase. Drying is needed for the following purposes:

(1) For the preparation of granules which can be dispensed in bulk, compressed in the form of tablets or filled in capsules.
(2) For the preparation of certain products like dried aluminium hydroxide, spray dried lactose and powdered extracts.
(3) For reducing the bulk and weight, thereby lowering the cost of transportation and storage.
(4) Vegetable drugs are dried before extraction to facilitate grinding and to avoid deterioration on storage.
(5) As dried products are more stable than moist ones therefore heat is required for drying.

Various methods and equipments for drying are available the choice of which depends on the following factors:

(i) Whether the product is sensitive to heat or not.
(ii) Physical characteristics of the product before drying.
(iii) The nature of the solvent to be removed.
(iv) Whether the process is to be carried out under aseptic conditions or not.
(v) Quantity of the product to be dried.
(vi) Available source of heat.
(viii) Cost involved.

Types of Dryers

(1) Dryers for dilute solutions, suspensions and slurries include:
   (a) Drum dryer
   (b) Spray dryer.
(2) Dryers for damp solid materials include:
   (a) Tray or shelf dryers.
   (b) Tunnel dryers.
   (c) Rotary dryer.
   (d) Fluidized bed dryer.
   (e) Vacuum dryer.
   (f) Freeze drying.

(1) Dryers for dilute solution, suspensions and slurries

(a) Drum dryer

Drum dryer consists of a steel drum 0.75 to 1.5 m in diameter and 2 to 4 m in length which is heated internally by steam and rotated on its longitudinal axis. The liquid to be dried is kept in a feeding pan in which the heated drum dips. As the drum rotates the liquid is applied to the surface and spreads to a film which dries rapidly. The dried product is scrapped from the surface of the drum by means of a doctor knife, in the form of flakes. The drying rate can be controlled by adjusting rotation speed and temperature of the drum.

Advantages

(i) It is a quick method of drying as the material spreads in a thin film over large surface area.

(ii) Heating time is short i.e. only a few seconds.

(iii) The equipment is compact which requires small space for its operation.

(iv) The equipment can be enclosed in a vacuum chamber thereby temperature of drying can be reduced.

(v) The product is obtained in flake form which has added advantages.

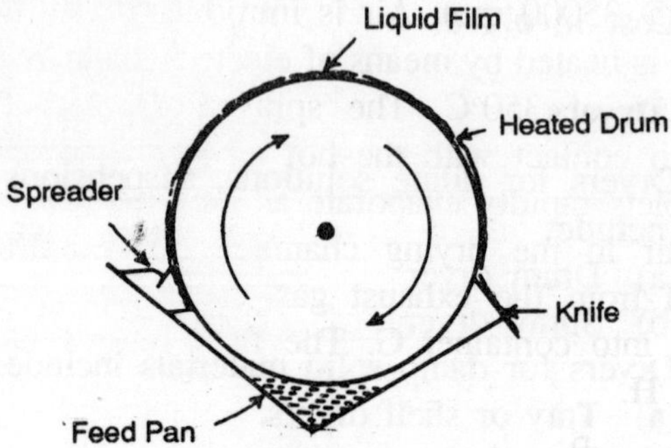

Fig. 12.1 Drum dryer

The substances which can be dried by this method include milk products, starch products, iron salts and suspensions of kaolin or zinc oxide etc.

(b) Spray dryer

Spray dryers are used for drying only the liquid materials such as solutions, slurries and thin pastes. In this method the liquid is dispersed as fine droplets into a moving stream of hot air where they are evaporated rapidly before reaching the wall of the chamber. The product dries into a fine powder which is collected into a collection system. There are many types of spray dryers designed to suit the material to be dried. All the spray dryers consists of the following components i.e. (i) feed delivery system, (ii) atomizer, (iii) heated air supply, (iv) drying chamber, (v) solid-gas separator, (vi) product collection system.

The material to be dried is fed to the atomizer D by gravity or by use of a suitable pump. The rate of feed is adjusted in such a way that each droplet of sprayed liquid is completely dried before it comes in contact with the walls of drying chamber and yet the dried powder is not overheated in the process. The inlet air temperature is kept constant. Too high a temperature can result in improper drying. Similarly excessive feed rates will lower the outer temperature due to which the material will be collected on the walls of the chamber. The disc of the atomizer D is driven by an air turbine and spins at @ 35000 rpm. Air is introduced with the help of fan B, which is heated by means of electric heater A to a maximum temperature of 350°C. The sprayed droplets from atomizer come into contact with the hot air just below the disc at C. The droplets rapidly evaporate as they are carried by currents of hot air in the drying chamber E. The dried powder is separated from the exhaust gas in cyclone separator F. and collected into container G. The flow rate of air is controlled by valve H.

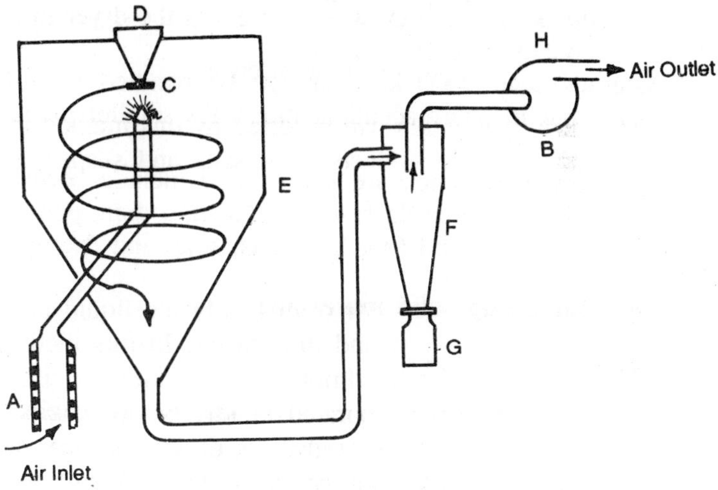

Fig. 12.2 Spray dryer

Applications

1. The material can be dried at a very fast rate. i.e. the actual drying time for a droplet is only a few seconds.
2. Since the evaporation rate is very high droplets are not subjected to a very high temperature.

3. The thermolabile substances can be easily dried without decomposition.
4. Spray dryers can be designed for drying under sterile conditions.
5. The dried powder will have a uniform particle size and shape.
6. Because of good flow properties the spray dried powders can be easily compressed in the form of tablets.
7. Labour costs are low since the material is dried in a single operation with no handling.

Disadvantages

1. The equipment is very bulky and costly. The drying chamber alone may be 15 m in height and 6 m in diameter.
2. There is lot of wastage of heat since the air must still be hot enough when it leaves the dryer to avoid condensation of moisture.

Materials upto 2000 kg/hour can be handled with large size plants but in pharmaceutical industries smaller plants are used.

The substances which are spray dried include boric acid, methyl cellulose, sulphur, lactose, citric acid, sodium phosphate, gelatin, acacia, milk and food products, soap and detergents.

2. Dryers for damp solid materials:

(a) Tray or shelf dryers

Tray or shelf dryers are also known as cabinet or compartment dryers. These types of dryers are essentially hot air ovens. The material to be dried is spread in thin layers in trays the number of which varies according to the size of the oven. The heating is done by the forced circulation of large volume of heated air by means of fans.

In truck dryers the trays are loaded on trucks (racks fitted with wheels) which can be pushed and taken out easily from the drying chamber. In pharmaceutical industries truck dryers are preferred over tray dryers because of convenience in loading and unloading the drying cabinets.

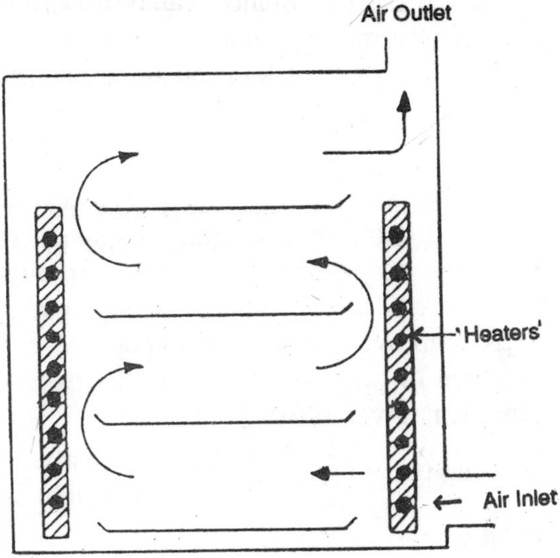

Fig. 12.3 Tray dryer

Drying by means of truck or tray dryers is a batch process rather than continuous drying as in the case of moving belt dryers. In pharmaceutical industries batch drying is preferred because each batch can be dried separately and same equipment can be used for drying a wide variety of materials.

(b) Tunnel dryers

Tunnel dryer is a modification of tray dryer in which oven is replaced by a tunnel. The material to be dried is entered at one end and the dried material is collected at the other end of the tunnel. The trays containing the wet material is loaded on trucks or on single or multiple belt conveyers which has an automatic speed control. In the multiple belt conveyer system the partially dried material which has completed one circle moves automatically from the end of the 1st conveyer on to the 2nd conveyer moving in the opposite direction. In this way the product may travel successively five times along the tunnel before it is discharged at the other end of the tunnel.

As compared to the tray dryers, the tunnel dryers have the advantage that it is semi-continuous as well as continuous in operation and can be used for large scale production.

(c) Rotary dryer

Rotary dryer is a modified form of tunnel dryer which consists of a horizontal tube, slightly inclined, so that the material fed at one end will move gradually through the tube towards the other end as the tube is slowly rotated at about 10 rev/min. To improve contact, the cylindrical tube is fitted with baffles which lift the solids and spill the particles through the air stream. This gives rapid drying.

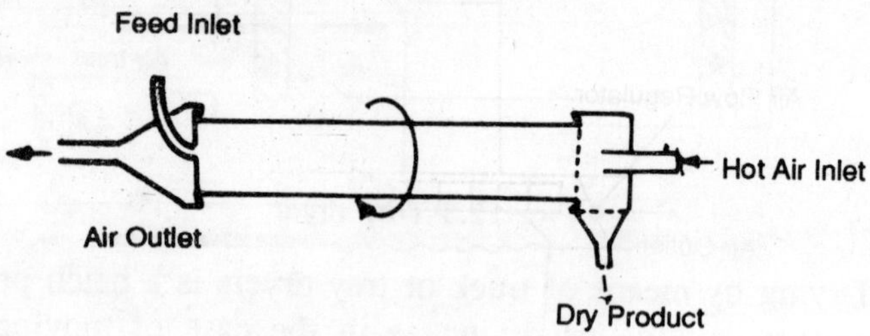

Fig. 12.4 Rotary dryer

Heating is done either directly, by a hot air current within the tube or indirectly through an outer shell containing steam tubes or heated gases. Due to the rotation of the cylinder, the material is turned over by tumbling effect and drying takes place from individual particles and not from static bed.

When recovery of solvent is important then rotary vacuum dryer may be used. Small rotary vacuum dryers are used for aseptic work. Such dryers are made up of stainless steel and all parts can be sterilized.

The rotary dryers are generally used for continuous drying of powdered or granular solids on large scale and several tonnes of material can be dried per hour.

(d) Fluidised bed dryer

Fluidised bed dryer is known by the name because a gas is allowed to flow upward through a bed of particulate solids at a velocity greater than the settling velocity of the particles, the solids will be blown up and become partially suspended in the gas stream. The resultant mixture of solids and gas behaves like a liquid and the solids are said to be fluidized. This technique is very efficient and is used for drying granular solids because each particle is surrounded by the drying gas.

Two types of fluidised bed dryers are used in pharmaceutical industries i.e. vertical and horizontal. The vertical type is used for batch drying whereas horizontal type is used for continuous drying. A typical vertical fluidised bed dryer for pharmaceutical use is shown in the diagram.

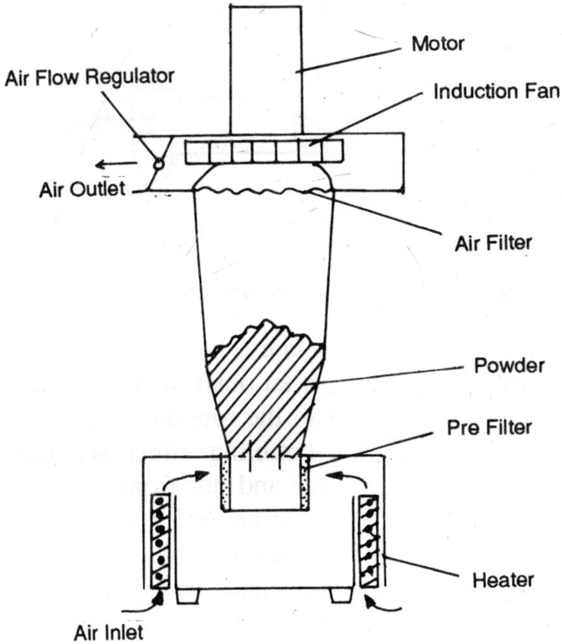

Fig. 12.5 Fluidized bed dryer

It consists of stainless steel chamber with a perforated bottom, into which the wet material to be dried is placed. For loading and unloading the drying chamber is removed from the unit. The air is introduced from below which is heated by means of heaters fitted therein, filtered and then passes through the powder bed by means of induction fan fitted in the upper part of the apparatus. The air is heated to the required temperature and its flow rate is adjusted. As the velocity of the air is increased, the bed begins to expand. Further increase in velocity beyond this point will cause rapid expansion of the bed and particles begin to show a turbulent motion "fluidisation". The particles are not in direct contact with each other and efficient heat exchange takes place between the particles and the flowing air. The moist air is carried away rapidly. With these types of dryers materials ranging from 5k g to 200 kg can be dried in about 20 to 40 minutes compared with 24 hour cycle in conventional tray dryers.

Advantages

1. They are efficient as material can be dried within 20 to 40 minutes compared with several hours in tray dryers.
2. Drying takes place from individual particles and not from whole bed.
3. The temperature of a fluidised bed is uniform and can be controlled to the desired temperature.
4. A free flowing product is produced.
5. Since the containers are mobile which make handling easy thereby labour costs are reduced.
6. Due to short drying time the unit has a high output

Disadvantages

1. Due to turbulence of the fluidised state, large quantities of fines are produced but the use of suitable binders during granulation can overcome this defect.
2. Too wet granules stick together on drying therefore too wet granules must not be used.
3. Many organic powders develop electrostatic charges during fluidisation so efficient electrical earthing of the drying chamber and the cloth filters is necessary.

Fluidised bed drier can be used for drying any powdered material but has special application in drying the tablet granules and is widely used for this purpose.

(e) Vacuum dryer

In pharmaceutical practice the vacuum oven is commonly used for vacuum drying. Vacuum oven is a modified form of vacuum still and consists of a jacketed vessel sufficiently hard in construction to withstand vacuum within the oven and steam pressure in the jacket. This type of oven is constructed in such a way that it provides large surface area for heat transfer by conduction and is provided with a door which can be tightly closed to provide air tight seal. The oven is connected through a condenser and receiver to a vacuum pump, the vacuum pump can be connected directly to the oven. For drying the material is spread on trays which are placed on steam heated shelves in the jacket of vacuum oven.

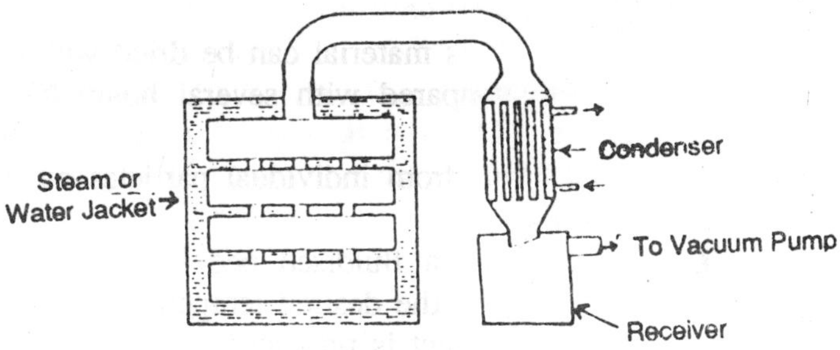

Fig. 12.6 Vacuum dryer

Advantages

(1) Thermolabile substances can be dried at a low temperature and chances of oxidation are reduced.

(2) During the manufacture of a dry extract, a porous and friable product is obtained which is especially useful in tablet manufacturing.

(3) By the use of condenser the solvent can be recovered from the product.

Disadvantages

(1) Heat transfer may be low and non uniform.

(2) The capacity of vacuum oven is limited therefore may not be suitable for large quantities.
(3) Labour and running costs are high.
(4) After drying a grinding process is necessary to get a powdered product.
(5) There is danger that the finally powdered material may be drawn off by the vacuum pump, and filters which require frequent cleaning have to be provided.

(f) Freeze drying

Freeze drying is the process in which water is removed from liquid products by sublimation hence this process is also known as sublimation drying. As the dried product has great affinity for water(lyophilic-liquid loving) therefore this process is also known as lyophilization. In this process the liquid is first frozen to ice before application of vacuum, to avoid frothing then sublimation of frozen ice is carried out under reduced pressure. The vaporization of ice occurs only at the surface hence the frozen ice is exposed to large surface area for rapid sublimation.

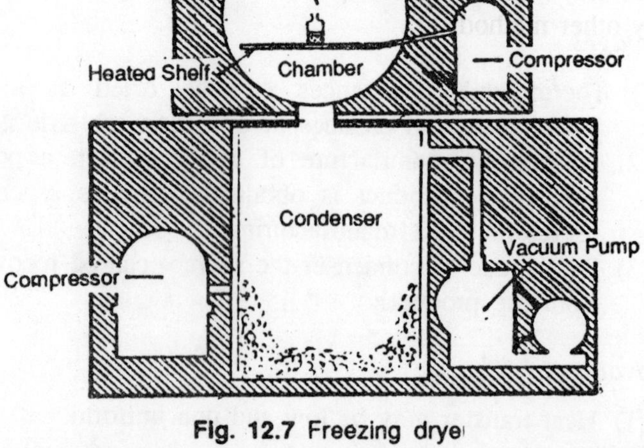

Fig. 12.7 Freezing dryer

Freeze drying on large scale may be carried out by freezing the product in a container kept on the shelf of a chamber by circulating a refrigerant like freon, ammonia or ethylene glycol from the compressor through the pipes fitted along the sides of the shelf. When the freezing is complete, vacuum is applied to the chamber which has been previously chilled by means of circulating the refrigerant from the large compressor.

Heat is then supplied to the product by heating coils or by circulating hot water. The process is continued till the product is dry and a spongy solid material is left behind.

The liquid products to be freeze dried are sterilized and distributed aseptically to the final containers which are kept open during the drying process and are immediately sealed as soon as the drying is complete.

Applications

Freeze drying is used for the manufacture of certain pharmaceutical and biological products which are thermolabile. It is also used for drying blood plasma, vitamins, enzymes, hormones and antibiotics.

Freeze dried product has definite physical properties as compared to products dried by other methods. Freeze-dried products are more stable than vacuum dried products and are often more readily soluble.

Since freeze-drying is very slow and expensive process it is preferably used for those products which cannot be dried by any other method.

13
Sterilization

Sterilization is the process of killing or removing bacteria and all other forms of living microorganisms and their spores from preparations or articles. A product is said to be sterile when it is free from all living microorganisms and passes the sterility tests.

13.1 Other Terms Used in Relation to Sterilization

Antiseptics : These are the substances used to inhibit the growth or destroy germs. They are used on the skin.

Bactericides : These are the substances used to kill bacteria.

Bacteriostatic Agents : These are the agents which inhibit the growth of bacteria. Different bacteriostatic agents are used against different bacteria.

Disinfectants : These are the agents used to kill bacteria and other infectious agents from the non-living articles. They are too strong to be applied to the human body.

Fungicides : These are the agents which kill fungi.

Germicides : These are the substances which kill germs but not necessarily bacterial spores.

Mycocides : These are the agents which kill molds.

Viricides : These are the agents which kill viruses.

The products or materials which require sterilization include all parenteral preparations including implants, ophthalmic preparations, surgical instruments, ligatures and sutures, surgical dressings, gloves etc. The working area where aseptic techniques are to be performed should also be sterilized.

13.2 Differences Between Sterilization and Disinfection

Sterilization differs from disinfection that in sterilization there is complete destruction or removal of all bacterial life including their spores but in disinfection there is destruction of bacterias but not their spores. It is not necessary that all the microorganisms are killed but their number is reduced to such an extent that they are not harmful to health. In other words it may be explained that in disinfection only the infe bacteria are destroyed. Generally the term disinfection is used to kill the microorganisms from inanimate objects and materials. The substances used in this way are known as disinfectants which include phenol, cresol, cresol with soap solution, chloroxylenol etc.

13.3 Thermal Resistance of Microorganisms

The microorganisms show varying resistance to sterilization procedures. The degree of resistance varies with the specific organisms particularly with spores of microorganisms which are more resistant than vegetative forms of the organism. Therefore before planning the sterilization process it must be ensured that the method and its conditions must be lethal to the resistant spores and the following points should be taken into consideration:

(a) Thermal death time

The thermal death time may be defined as the time required to kill a specific type of microorganism at a given temperature under specified conditions. It not only depends on controllable factors like temperature, pH, presence of bactericide etc but also depends on uncontrollable factors such as number of contaminating microorganisms and their resistance to heat.

The table 13.1 shows approximate values of thermal death times of different spores to moist heat and dry heat.

Table 13.1 Approximate thermal death times of different spores

	Time in minutes					
	Moist heat			Dry heat		
Organism	100°C	110°C	121°C	120°C	140°C	170°C
1. B.anthracis	5-15	-	-	-	180	-
2. Cl.welchii	5-10	-	-	50	5	-
3. Cl.tetani	5-15	-	-	-	15	-
4. Cl.botulinum	330	90	10	120	60	15
5. Soil bacilli	>1020	120	6	-	-	15

It will be seen from the above table that there is a considerable variation in thermal death times between different types of bacterial spores therefore an adequate margin of safety should be kept to kill the most resistant species of microorganisms and spores expected to be present by exceeding temperature and time for which it is applied than the known thermal death times of most of the spores. Commonly the thermal death time indicated is increased by 50 percent.

(b) Death rate of microorganisms

By direct method it is not possible to determine that when the sterility is first achieved because shortly before sterility is reached the number of living organisms is so small that accurate determination of it becomes impossible due to very high errors in taking the samples. Therefore reliable method is to plot a graph of log survivors against time of exposure.

(c) Decimal reduction time (D value)

It is one of the functions to indicate the efficiency of sterilization process. This is the time in minutes required to reduce the number of viable organisms by 90 percent i.e. the time corresponding to one log cycle on the survivor/time curve. The order of death of microorganisms can be calculated from the equation:

$$K = 1/t\ (\log No - \log N)$$

where K is constant depending on the organism, temperature, medium and assuming logarithms to the base 10; it is the time of exposure in minutes; No is the number of organisms viable at the beginning of the time interval and N is the number of organisms viable at the end of the time interval.

It was noted that after 90% reduction in microorganisms the following equation was obtained:

$$\begin{aligned} K &= 1/t\ (\log No - \log 0.1\ No) \\ &= 1/t\ (\log No - \log 10^{-1}\ No) \\ &= 1/t\ [\log No - (\log 10^{-1} + \log No)] \\ &= 1/t\ [\log No - (-1) \log 10 - \log No] \\ &= 1/t\ (1) \log 10 \\ &= 1/t \\ t &= 1/k \end{aligned}$$

Time t was defined as the decimal reduction time which is called the D value.

$$D = 1/k$$

The value of D can be found out by calculating K from the graph of logarithm of the number of surviving organisms against time of exposure.

13.4. Factors Affecting the Thermal Destruction of Microorganisms

The following factors affect the thermal destruction of microorganisms:

1. pH
2. Inhibitory medicaments
3. Antibacterial agents
4. Protective substances
5. Initial number of organisms
6. The inactivation factor of the process.

1. pH

Most of microorganisms are resistant to heat at a pH of 6 to 8, therefore acidic or alkaline solutions are easier to sterilize. Certain substances like alkaloidal salts which act as buffers for acidic or alkaline pH may be used for preserving stability. Such conditions help in the sterilization of an injection.

2. Inhibitory medicaments

Certain medicaments in solution form are harmful to microorganisms. In certain cases it is due to pH but in others the medicament itself is toxic. Although some of the non-sporing microorganisms e.g. Staphylococcus aureus are killed within 24 hours at room temperature by a number of medicaments in their usual strength but spores are not killed unless they are heated to sterilizing conditions of time and temperature. Therefore very few injections can be safely regarded as self-sterilizing.

3. Antibacterial agents

The addition of antibacterial agents in injections can reduce the sterilizing temperature from 115°C to 100°C which is quite useful in relatively thermolabile substances and the sterilization methods so used is known as sterilization by heating with a bactericide

4. Protective substances

In media containing high concentrations of organic substances such as proteins and carbohydrates the micro-organisms are not easily killed, the reasons are not clearly understood but it is believed protein forms a protective coat on the cells.

Since most protein containing injections are heat sensitive therefore cannot be sterilized by heat hence do not create much problem but this effect is found in injections containing thermostable carbohydrates such as dextrose which is used in very high concentrations i.e. upto 50 percent. However it has been seen that any increase in resistance of organisms is over-come by normal sterilizing conditions.

This problem is more important in sterilization of equipment such as tubes, syringes, containers etc. which are not thoroughly cleaned after use for proteins like blood or blood products etc. or carbohydrates such as dextrose etc because some of the microorganisms may remain hidden inside the equipment and protected from steam. Therefore thorough cleaning of equipment is very important.

5. Initial number of organisms

When a certain number of organisms are heated at a lethal temperature, the organisms are not killed all atonce but they are killed gradually as the exposure is prolonged. If certain fraction of initial number is destroyed in a particular time interval then the same fraction will be destroyed in the succeeding interval of time and will continue till all the organisms are killed and the preparation is sterilized e.g. with an initial number of 10^6/ml and a death rate of 90 percent/min, the number surviving after each of the first six minutes will be 10^5,10^4,10^3,10^2,10 and 1 per ml respectively. This is known as exponential or logarithmic death rate. If the number of survivors (in unit volume) are plotted against time a smooth curve is obtained but if logarithms of this number are plotted then a straight line is produced.

From the above figures it is clear that if the initial number of organisms is less, then the time required for sterilization will be less. Therefore as far as possible thoroughly cleaned containers and equipment should be used and precautions should be taken to eliminate the entry of organisms to solutions during their preparation. This will facilitate the sterilization process.

6. The inactivation factor of the process

The inactivation factor is the degree to which the viable population of organisms is reduced and is obtained by dividing the initial viable count by the final viable count otherwise if D value for the organism is known it can be calculated as follows:

Inactivation factor = 10 t/D where t is the exposure time in minutes and D is the decimal reduction time for the same temperature and conditions.

13.5. Methods of Sterilization

Methods of sterilization have been divided into following ategories:

1. Physical Methods

(a) Dry heat sterilization.
(b) Moist heat sterilization (steam sterilization).
(c) Sterilization by radiations.

2. Chemical Methods

(a) Gaseous sterilization.
(b) Sterilization by disinfectants.

3. Mechanical Methods

In these methods of sterilization the solution to be sterilized is passed through a mechanical device known as bacteria proof filter which include millipore filter, Setiz filter, sintered glass filter, Berkefeld filter etc.

Several factors are important in killing bacteria which include temperature, pH of the solution, presence of bactericidal chemicals, presence or absence of moisture, carbohydrates or proteins.

The most suitable temperature for the growth of pathogenic microorganisms is 37°C. Most vegetative bacterias are killed by heating at 60°C for 10 minutes in the presence of moisture. However spores are much more resistant and require special methods of sterilization for their destruction.

The methods used in attaining sterility in a pharmaceutical preparation is determined largely by the nature of the preparation and its ingredients. However regardless of the methods used for sterilization, the final product must pass a test for sterility. Moist heat is more effective than dry heat sterilization but moist heat under pressure is the most suitable method for sterilization of solutions or liquid preparations and should be preferably used wherever applicable.

1. Physical Methods

(a) Dry Heat Sterilization

Substances which get destroyed by moist heat or due to their physical characteristics cannot be sterilized by moist heat may be sterilized by dry heat in ovens designed specially for this purpose which are electrically heated and thermostatically controlled.

Substances which are sterilized by dry heat include fixed oils, glycerin, liquid paraffin, petrolatum, propylene glycol and powders such as talc or zinc oxide. In addition, dry heat sterilization is the method of choice for sterilization of glassware, many surgical instruments and surgical catgut. Preparations containing water, alcohol or other volatile substances and surgical dressings cannot be sterilized by this method because at high temperature liquids may evaporate and dressing may char.

During dry heat sterilization the microorganisms and bacterial spores are killed by oxidation. Since dry heat is less effective than moist heat, higher temperatures and longer periods of exposure are required. Exposure at 160°C for 1 hour is required for dry heat sterilization. The exposure time depends on packaging of the material, thickness of glass, volume of container etc. for example syringes and needles may be sterilized at 160°C for 1 hour but glycerin or liquid paraffin must be sterilized at 160°C for 2 hour or at 170°C for 1 hour. Consequently higher temperatures require shorter exposure time for a given substance and on the other hand lower temperatures require longer exposure time. A substance which gets decomposed at a higher temperature may be sterilized at low temperature exposed for long period of time. Dry heat sterilization may be done by means of direct flame (flaming) or by hot air oven.

(a) Flaming

Flaming is the simplest method of dry heat sterilization in which the material to be sterilized is kept in the hot part of Bunsen burner's flame for a few seconds and the process is repeated several times. This method is generally used for those articles which are to be used immediately e.g. forceps, needles, knives, blades, scalpels, metal spatulas, the mouth of culture tubes and bottles, and platinum loops. This method is not reliable for sterilizing greasy or oily materials.

(b) Hot-air Oven

Hot air oven or dry heat sterilizer consists of a metallic chamber of aluminium or stainless steel, which is electrically heated and thermostatically controlled. There are two types of ovens (1) in which air is circulated by gravity convection to all parts of the chamber (2) "mechanical convection type" in which air is circulated by a fan. The latter type is more satisfactory because the sterilizing temperature is more readily controlled.

The chamber of the oven has double walls which are separated from each other by thick layer of glass-fibre insulation. The hollow flanged door is also filled with glass fibre insulation. The inner side of the door is fitted with asbestos gasket that provides a tight seal to prevent heat loss. Depending on the size of the oven 3-4 perforated shelves are provided in the chamber which can be removed as and when desired. A good quality thermometer is fitted in front of the chamber for noting the temperature during the process. A fan is provided for air circulation in the oven. A vent is fitted at the top of the oven. An on-off switch is provided along with green and red indicators. The heating elements are fitted on the lower side of chamber. Heat is transferred from the source to the articles by conduction, convection and radiation.

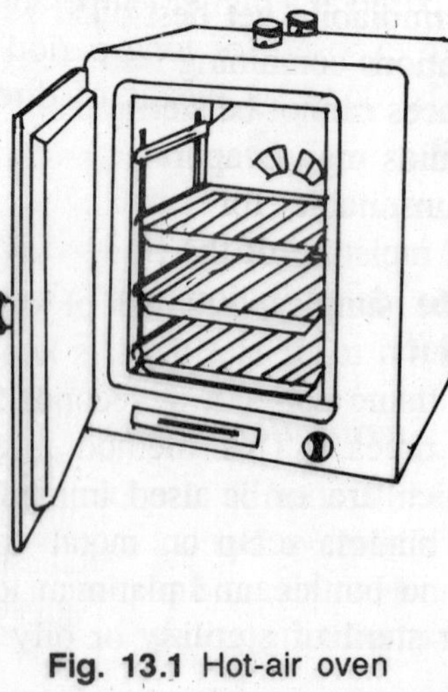

Fig. 13.1 Hot-air oven

For getting good results the oven should be properly loaded so that all the articles are exposed to uniform heat for required time. Care should be taken that the oven is not opened in between the sterilization operation. Glasswares (thoroughly cleaned and dried) like conical flasks, test tubes, pipettes etc. should be plugged with non-absorbent cotton wool because absorbent cotton wool becomes saturated during sterilization and the plugs act as inefficient seals because the motile bacteria can swim through the attached moisture into the tubes.

Advantages of Dry-Heat Sterilization

1. It is most suitable method of sterilization for substances which are destroyed by moisture e.g. oily substances and dry powders.
2. Glasswares like flasks, test tubes, pipettes, all glass syringes etc. can be easily and thoroughly sterilized which may not be possible in moist heat sterilization.
3. It is less damaging to glass and metal equipment than moist heat.

Disadvantages of Dry-Heat Sterilization

1. It requires very long heating up times, high temperature and long exposure time.
2. Most medicaments, rubber and plastic articles which are thermolabile get destroyed by this method.
3. Preparations containing water, alcohol or other volatile substances cannot be sterilized by this method because the liquids may evaporate at high temperature.
4. It is unsuitable for surgical dressings because the natural moisture of the fibres quickly vaporises which leads to deterioration and ultimately charring may take place.

(b) Moist Heat Sterilization

Moist heat sterilization is also known as steam sterilization. It is done in an autoclave but on small scale a pressure cooker can be used, in which steam under pressure is used. It is the most reliable method of sterilization because in the presence of moisture bacteria are destroyed at a considerably lower temperature rather than when moisture is absent. In fact, bacterial cells with a large percentage of water are killed easily. Spores, which contain relatively low percentage of water are comparatively difficult to kill. By this method the microorganisms are destroyed by denaturation and coagulation of some of the essential proteins present in the microorganisms. Moist heat sterilization is more powerful than dry heat sterilization because (a) the penetrating power of steam is much more than that of dry heat (b) the thermal capacity of steam is much greater than that of dry heat (c) in presence of moisture, denaturation or coagulation of essential proteins present in microorganisms takes place at lower temperature.

(1) **Autoclaving** Autoclaving is the process of heating in an autoclave in which saturated steam under pressure is allowed to penetrate through the materials for at least 15 minutes at a minimum temperature of 121°C. The measurement of time begins when the temperature of the material being sterilized reaches 121°C. It should be noted that it is the temperature which destroyes the micro-organisms and not the pressure, the pressure helps in increasing the temperature of the system.

The following table shows the relationship between pressure and temperature and the exposure times commonly employed for sterilization by steam under pressure.

Pressure	*Temperature*	*Time*
10 pounds	115.5°C	30 minutes
15 pounds	121.5°	20 minutes
20 pounds	126.5°	15 minutes

From the above table it is clear that greater the pressure applied, higher the temperature obtained and lesser the time required for sterilization. Generally the sterilization in an autoclave is done at a temperature of 121°C for 15 minutes.

Autoclave is an apparatus used for sterilization by steam under pressure. A portable or bench autoclave is quite similar to pressure cooker. It is a hollow cylindrical vessel of about 15 litres capacity made up of aluminium or stainless steel, fitted with a lid which can be firmly secured. In one type of

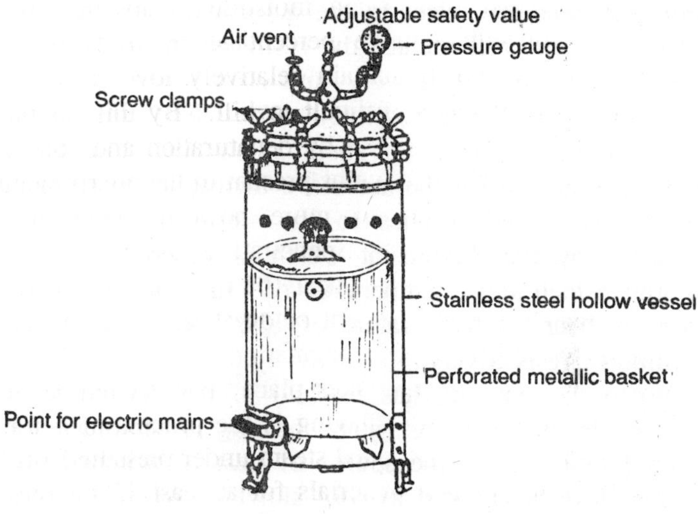

Fig. 13.2 Autoclave

autoclave the lid is fitted with eight screw clamps, a pressure gauge, an air vent and an adjustable safety valve. The externally fitted lid has the advantage that whole of the capacity of the vessel can be used but at the same time it has disadvantage also that even if one clamp is damaged or left loose, the pressure imposed on others may lead to explosion. Therefore it is essential that all the clamps should be firmly secured and should be carefully maintained. The autoclave is electrically heated, the electric elements are fitted at the bottom of the autoclave. It is provided with a perforated metallic basket fitted with legs, in which the material to be sterilized is placed.

Working

The working of this type of autoclave is very simple. The perforated metallic basket is taken out of the vessel and a bucket full of water is put in the vessel so that the heating elements get completely immersed in water. The material to be sterilized is loosely packed in the basket which is then kept in the autoclave. Care should be taken that the basket should not touch the water. The lid is tightly fitted in position and the source of heat switched on, air vent it kept open.

After sometime the water in the autoclave starts boiling and steam generated will replace the entire air in the body of the autoclave (this factor is very important otherwise complete sterilization may not be possible). When the steam has passed freely through the vent for about 5 minutes, close the vent. As the pressure inside the autoclave increases, the temperature also increases and reaches to the sterilizing point already controlled by the thermostat which is generally 10 pounds per square inch and a temperature of 115°C or 15 pounds per square inch and a temperature of 121°C for 30 minutes and 20 minutes respectively.

When the pressure has reached to the desired level, as indicated by the pressure gauge, heating is continued for the required time. Then the source of heat is switched off and the autoclave is allowed to cool slowly. When the pressure inside and outside the autoclave equals or drops to zero level, the steam vent is opened and lid removed to take out the sterilized material.

(2) **Horizontal Large Scale Autoclave** The portable autoclaves described above can only be used for small number of articles or for a few transfusion bottles. On larger scale e.g. In hospitals and industries horizontal autoclaves are used which may measure upto 20 ft in length and 12 inch to 6 ft in diameter. In pharmaceutical industries, double door autoclaves are used in which the substances to be sterilized are introduced through one door and taken out through the other door. The construction and working of horizontal autoclaves are basically the same as that of portable autoclaves but steam may be introduced from an outer source.

Advantages of Moist Heat Sterilization

1. Because of high penetration power of steam under pressure, microorganisms are killed more efficiently and in lesser time at low temperatures than dry heat.
2. In large size autoclaves large quantities of materials can be sterilised in one batch.
3. Solutions packed in sealed containers, as ampoules, are readily sterilized by this method.

4. Bulk solutions, glassware, surgical dressings, rubber gloves and surgical instruments are effectively sterilized by this method.

Disadvantages of Moist Heat Sterilization

1. This method is unsuitable for materials which cannot withstand the heating at 115°C or more.
2. This method is not useful for oils, fats, ointments, powders, oily injections; and other preparations through which steam cannot penetrate.

(3) **Heating with a Bactericide** This is a special method of moist heat sterilization at 100°C which is used for sterilizing aqueous solutions and suspensions that are destroyed by high temperatures of autoclaving. A bactericide in suitable proportion is added to the solutions to be sterilized which is distributed in final containers and sealed. The sealed containers are then heated at 100°C at 30 minutes in a steam sterilizer or water bath. This method is based on the fact that killing is done by heat as well as by bactericide, rather bactericides are more effective at high temperatures than at low temperatures.

The most commonly used bactericides include benzalkonium chloride 0.01%, chlorocresol 0.2%, phenylmercuric acetate 0.002% and phenylmercuric nitrate 0.002%.

The method should not be used for intravenous injections when a single does of the solution is more than 15 ml. Similarly preparations meant for intrathecal and intracisternal injections should not be prepared by this method.

(4) **Sterilization by boiling water at atmospheric pressure** The boiling water bath or electric boiling water sterilizer is most useful for sterilizing instruments like syringes, needles, knives, blades, scalpels, scissors and other surgical instruments. They should be completely dipped in boiling water and should be boiled at least for 20 minutes. After sterilization the materials should be removed with forceps already sterilized by dipping in suitable disinfectant or by heating in flame.

(5) **Other methods of sterilization** Other methods of sterilization include :

(i) Tyndallization or fractional sterilization.

(ii) *Pasterurization* Holding method and high temperature short time method.

These two methods has little advantage therefore they are not used now a days in pharmacy.

(6) **Moist heat sterilization at 55 to 60°C** This method is quite useful for sterilization of certain vaccines which get destroyed at a temperature higher than 60°C. The sealed containers containing the vaccine are immersed in a water bath which is thermostatically controlled. They are heated at 55-60°C for 15-60 minutes, depending on the nature of microorganisms to be killed. By this method the antigenic properities of the vaccines are protected whereas the bacteria are killed.

(c) Sterilization by Radiations

Sterilization by radiations is also known as "cold sterilization" because no heat is used in this method. The microorganisms are very susceptible to the lethal effects of ionizing radiations. The exact mechanism by which the microorganisms are destroyed is not clear. According to one theory alteration of chemicals presents in microorganisms takes place with the formation of new compounds which destroy the microorganisms. According to another theory the vital structures of cells, such as nucleoproteins are destroyed by which the microorganisms are killed.

Radiations may be classified as :

1. Electromagnetic waves which include infra-red radiations, ultraviolet light, X-ray and gamma rays.
2. Stream of minute particles of matter which includes alpha radiations and beta radiations also known as alpha particles and beta particles respectively.

Out of the above mentioned radiations only the infra-red radiations, ultraviolet light, gamma rays and high velocity electrons are used for sterilization. The other radiations are not used for sterilization purposes.

(1) **Ultra-violet light** Direct sunlight is quite harmful to the microorganisms, it can destroy them due to the presence of ultra violet rays in it. U.V. rays of shorter wavelengths are

more destructive than rays of longer wavelengths. These two types of rays are emitted by the sun. The rays of shorter wavelength are absorbed by the atmosphere where as rays of longer wavelength which are less harmful reach to the earth .

The penetration power of U.V. rays is very less, they are effective only to the exposed surface. Therefore they are commonly employed to reduce airborne contamination and sterilization of aseptic rooms or areas where the pharmaceutical processing is to be carried out. It is of little value as a sterilizing agent.

The most common source of artificial U.V. rays is the U.V. lamps by which U.V. radiations in the region of 2537 Å are produced which has germicidal activities. They are often used in pharmaceutical industries for sterilization of aseptic rooms and for naked surfaces such as table tops etc; for this purpose the lamps may be fitted at the top of the surface to be sterilized.

U.V. rays are very harmful to the skin and eyes therefore these organs must be properly protected by wearing hoods, gowns with long sleeves and rubber gloves. Eyes should be protected by wearing eyeshields e.g. plastic face masks.

(2) **Gamma Rays** Gamma rays are generally obtained from radio-active isotopes of cobalt 60. When the unstable atoms of this isotope disintegrate, they emit two gamma rays in succession. They kill microorganisms by ionization of atoms of essential substances present in the living cells of microorganisms.

Gamma rays are similar in nature to X-rays of short wavelength. Being electromagnetic radiations both of them have high penetration power, the fact which is used in sterilization.

Advantages of gamma radiation sterilization

1. Because of high penetration power these radiations are used in the preservation of foods. In pharmaceutical industries they are a satisfactory method of sterilization for parenteral preparations containing antibiotics like benzyl penicillin, streptomycin sulphate, polymixin

sulphate; vitamins like ascorbic acid; surphonamides such as sulphapyridine and sulphathiazole etc.

2. These radiations are used for sterilization of some bacterial and viral vaccines e.g. influenza, poliomyelitis and rabies vaccines.
3. There is no significant rise in temperature.
4. The process is continuous because short exposure time is required and a large quantity of material can be sterilized at once.
5. No aseptic handling is required because sterilization can be done after packing the material in final containers.
6. This method is quite reliable.

Disadvantages

1. Because of high cost involved, all the industries cannot afford to instal the plant.
2. These radiations are harmful to the persons engaged in this work so they must by protected and kept under constant attention.
3. They may lead to change in colour, solubility and texture of the preparation and may also lead to decomposition of certain medicaments.

2. Chemical Methods

(a) Gaseous Sterilization

Gaseous sterilization is a special type of chemical sterilization in which the chemicals used are gases or vapours and not the liquids or solids dissolved in a solution. Many gases like, sulphur dioxide, chlorine, ozone, formaldehyde, beta-propiolactone and ethylene oxide have bactericidal effects. Although formaldehyde was extensively used as a fumigant but now its use has found limited acceptance. Now a days ethylene oxide has become the most widely used gaseous sterilizing agent in pharmacy and medicine.

The gases used for chemical sterilization are as follows:

(1) **Ethylene oxide** Ethylene oxide is a colourless gas at ordinary temperature. It is a simple cyclic ether having the formula

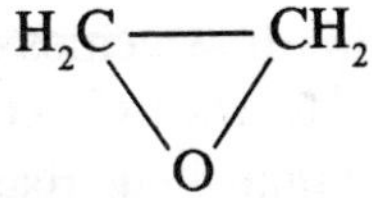

It is highly inflammable when mixed with air in concentrations more than 3% but when properly diluted with an inert gas such as carbon dioxide or a suitable flourinated hydrocarbon it becomes non-inflammable and can be safely used for sterilization purpose. A mixture of 90% carbon dioxide and 10% ethylene oxide are non-explosive and are commercially available.

The mode of action of ethylene oxide to kill the microorganisms is based on the process of alkylation of essential substances present in a protein molecule.

Sterilization by ethylene oxide is a complex process as compared to dry heat and moist heat sterilization because it requires greater precautions with regard to ethylene oxide concentration, temperature, humidity and time. Concentrations of ethylene oxide used for sterilization range from 200 to 1000 mg/litre. If the concentration is doubled the exposure time is reduced to half. Similarly with slight rise in temperature the sterilizing efficiency of ethylene oxide is increased which helps in the reduction of exposure time. In general the concentration of ethylene oxide used should be 450 mg/litre of sterilizer chamber space and must be exposed from 6 to 16 hours at temperatures of 49 to 60°C. However, if the materials to be sterilized are unable to withstand this slight rise in temperature, they should be sterilized at room temperature but exposed for longer periods.

Table 13.2

Ethylene oxide concentration	*Exposure time at 25°C*
88 mg/litre	10 hours
442 mg/litre	4 hours
884 mg/litre	2 hours

Gas sterilization requires specialized equipment which resembles autoclaves. The sterilizing chambers are fitted with an efficient vacuum pump, a control system to regulate the introduction of the gas mixture and to maintain the desired gas pressure, a device to control the humidity in the chamber and thermostatically controlled heating elements.

Advantages of Ethylene Oxide Sterilization

1. Thermolabile substances can be sterilized at room temperature or at a slightly raised temperature.
2. It has great penetrating power therefore quite useful for sterilizing surgical instruments such as catheters, needles and plastic disposable syringes.
3. It do not damage the moisture sensitive substances and equipments, rather, it needs moisture for killing the microorganisms. In anhydrous conditions it is not effective.
4. Powders packed in polythene bags can be sterilized by it.

Disadvantages of Ethylene Oxide Sterilization

1. Since it is a slow process therefore it requires long exposures, hence, unsuitable in emergencies.
2. Costly equipment is required for sterilization.
3. Since it is highly inflammable therefore requires special precautions.

Ethylene oxide sterilization is more expensive but less reliable than moist heat sterilization therefore it should not be used when the latter is practicable. For thermolabile substances ionizing radiations should be preferred than ethylene oxide for sterilization of articles required in bulk e.g. disposable syringes, needles, gloves, catheters etc.

(2) **Formaldehyde** It has been quite commonly used for fumigating the rooms and blankets used in the hospitals. It is quite effective bactericidal agent and kills all bacteria including spores. It is quite irritant and pungent in nature and has low penetrating power. Formaldehyde has been used in an alcoholic solution for disinfection of instruments.

Formaldehyde as sterilizing agent has disadvantages of low penetrating power through covered surfaces and it is difficult to expel the gas from the sterilizing area.

(3) **Beta-propiolactone (BPL)** It is a heterocyclic ring compound having the following formula

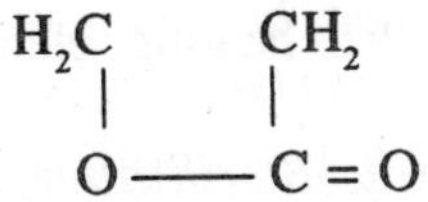

It is quite active at low concentrations hence used in concentrations of 2-5 mg/litre of space at 25°C. The BPL vapours are 5 times more active than formaldehyde vapours and 4000 times more active than ethylene oxide. It has low penetrating power, therefore used for sterilizing large areas such as laboratories and aseptic rooms. It is not used in pharmaceutical applications.

(b) Sterilization by Disinfectants

Disinfectants are mainly used for sterilizing the surfaces used for aseptic work. In emergency they may be used for sterilizing the surgical instruments like forceps, scissors, knives, blades etc. For this purpose the required instruments may be dipped in the disinfectant and afterwards washed with sterilized water. The commonly used disinfectants include: alcohol, iodine, isopropyl alcohol , chlorine, cresol with soap solution, phenol and formaldehyde.

3. Mechanical Methods

(a) Sterilization by filtration

Sterilization by filtration is one of the oldest methods of sterilization used in pharmacutical industries for small scale filtration operations. In this method the solutions to be sterilized are passed through bacteria proof filters which include Berkefeld, Pasteur-Chamberland, Seitz and Millipore filters. This method is very useful for thermolabile solutions and can also be used for other solutions. The microorganisms are physically removed by adsorption on the filter medium or by a sieving mechanism. The bacterias are entrapped in the pores of the filters and are removed from the solution. Since the filtration through these pores is very slow, vacuum and/or pressure are employed to enhance the filtration. In practice, the filter, the accessories, and the receiving vessels must be sterilized by suitable means and kept sterile throughout the operation. This method requires, that aseptic conditions must be maintained. The apparatus should be thoroughly inspected before use for cracks or breakage which may render it unfit for sterilization purposes. After passing the solution through bacteria proof filters it is distributed into sterile containers, under aseptic conditions. The containers are then sealed.

Although all the processes i.e. filtration, filling and sealing are done under aseptic conditions but still the microorganisms may enter into the solution from atmosphere or containers, therefore sterility tests must be performed on the filled containers.

13.6 Types of Filters

Various types of filters used for sterilizing the solutions by filtration are:

1. Seitz filter.
2. Sintered glass filters.
3. Berkefeld and Mandler filters.
4. Pasteur-Chamberland filters.
5. Millipore filters.
6. Membrane filters.

1. Seitz Filter

Seitz filter was developed in Germany and marketed under the trade name Seitz. They are usually round but occasionally square. These filters consist of two parts. The lower part is fitted with a perforated plate over which a compressed asbestos pad is placed which acts as a filtering media. The asbestos filter pads are made in several porosities out of which grade E.K. is used for bacterial filtration. The upper part has a valve through which pressure can be applied. The two parts i.e. upper and lower are joined together by means of winged nuts. The solution to be filtered is filled in the apparatus, pressure is applied through the valve and filtered solution is collected at the bottom in sterilized containers.

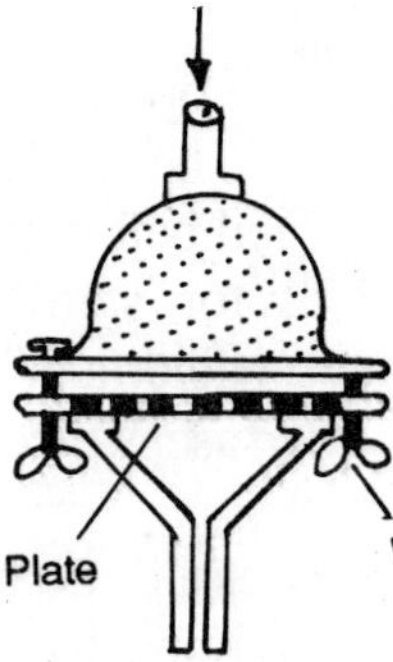

Fig. 13.3 Seitz filter

Advantages

1. As the pads are meant for single use , a new pad is to be used each time and there is no risk of contaminating the filtrate.
2. The apparatus is very simple to use.
3. For viscous solutions they are more suitable than ceramic or glass filters.

Disadvantages

1. Asbestos pads may shed loose fibres which makes the solutions unsuitable for injections.
2. It imparts alkalinity to the filtrate which may be sufficient to precipitate the alkaloids from solutions of their salts.
3. The pads may adsorb sufficient amount of medicament which may result in loss of volume specially when the quantity of solution is small.

2. Sintered Glass Filters

Sintered glass filters consist of ground glass particles which are fused together by heating to its sintering point (it is that temperature at which the glass particles are fused together to become solid, without melting). The fused particles have interstices between themselves which form a suitable system for filtration. They are prepared in the from of discs of suitable size and shape which are then sealed by heat in to a Pyrex glass funnel, having the shape of buchner funnel. These so fused funnels are known as sintered glass funnels, which are made in several porosities. For bacterial filtration Grade 5 having the maximum pore size of 2 µm is used, for clarification of solutions filters with other porosities are used.

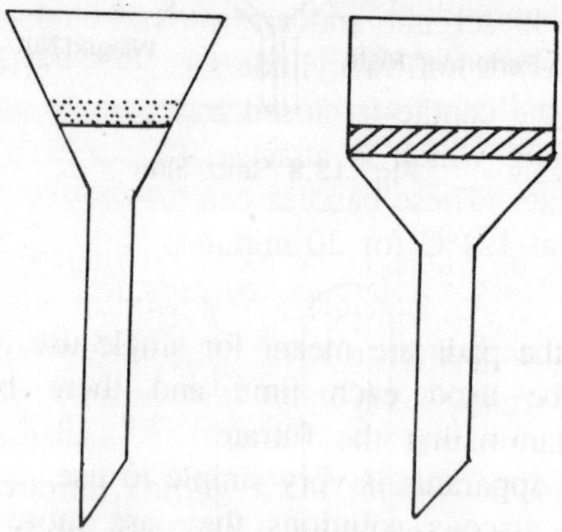

Fig. 13.4 Sintered glass filter

These filters are very fragile, so must be handled carefully. After use they must be cleaned thoroughly. For cleaning they must be washed by suction with hot hydrochloric acid and then with distilled water, until the medium is free from acid.

Advantages

1. If properly cleaned, nothing can enter into the filtrate therefore they are generally used for the filtration of solutions to be injected.
2. They are useful for filtering small as well as large volumes.
3. Very little amount of medicament may be absorbed.
4. Volume of filtrate retained in the medium is negligible.

Disadvantages

1. They are very costly.
2. The medium is unsuitable for large volume filtration because for this purpose large discs are required which are mechanically weak.

3. Berkefeld Filters

Berkefeld filters are test tube shaped filters called "filter candles" or "ceramic candles". They are made up of unglazed porcelain or kieselguhr and are available in various porosity grades. They are hollow cylinders mounted on metallic joints. One end of the candle is closed and the other is fitted with a narrow opening which is attached to a vacuum pump at the time of its use. These candles can be sterilized by moist heat sterilization at 121°C for 20 minutes.

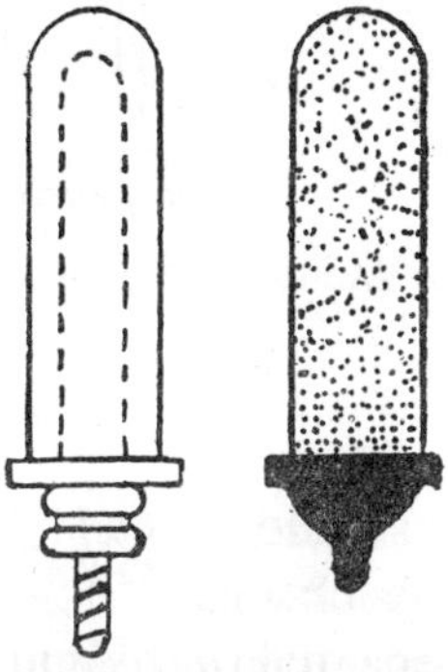

Fig. 13.5 Berkefeld filter

For filtration, the candle is placed in the solution to be sterilized. The narrow opening is attached to the vacuum pump. When the vacuum is applied and pressure inside the candle is decreased, the solution is forced to move inside the candle from where it is collected in large size sterilized containers. The solution so filtered is distributed in final containers which are sealed immediately. The whole process of filtration is carried out under strict aseptic conditions.

By the repeated use of filtration candles, they may get clogged and can be easily cleaned by scrubbing the outer surface of the filter with a brush and passing the water under pressure from inside to outside direction which will remove the entangled particles from the interstices.

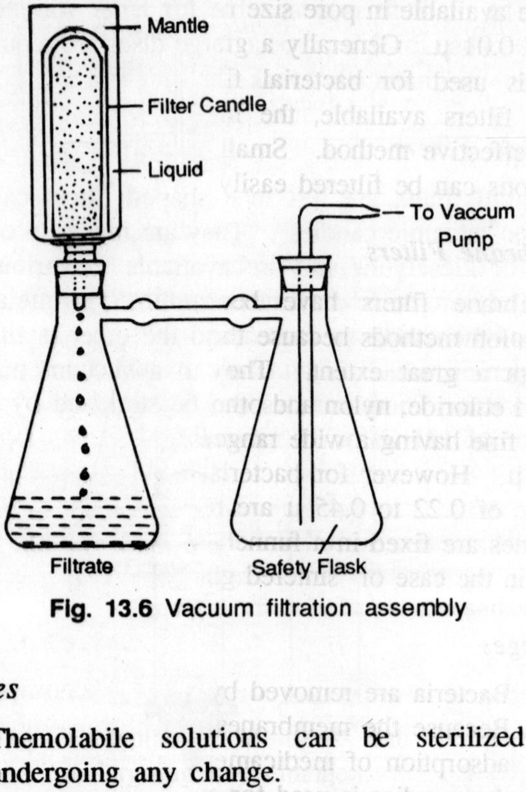

Fig. 13.6 Vacuum filtration assembly

Advantages

1. Themolabile solutions can be sterilized without undergoing any change.
2. All, living as well as dead microorganisms are removed.

Disadvantages

1. The main disadvantage of such filters is that the pores get blocked which require thorough cleaning before the process is repeated.
2. As compared to other filtration medias these candles are little difficult to fit into the filtration units.

4. Millipore Filters

They are porous structures made up of pure and biologically inert cellulose ester. These filters posses high degree of uniform pore size, high flow and high thermal stability. They do not absorb the solution and are resistant to chemicals. Millipore filters are available in pore size ranging from a high of 8 μ to a low of 0.01 μ. Generally a grade with pore size of 0.22 ± 0.02 μ is used for bacterial filtration. Among the various bacterial filters available, the millipore filters are the most suitable effective method. Small volumes and large volumes of solutions can be filtered easily.

5. *Membrane Filters*

Membrane filters have become very common among ultrafiltration methods because the membranes used have been refined to a great extent. They are made up of cellulose, polyvinyl chloride, nylon and other cellulose derivatives. They are very fine having a wide range of pore size from 8 μ down to 0.22 μ. However for bacterial filtration, membranes with pore size of 0.22 to 0.45 μ are recommended. For use these membranes are fixed in a funnel of desired size and shape as is done in the case of sintered glass funnels.

Advantages

1. Bacteria are removed by sieving.
2. Because the membranes used are very thin therefore adsorption of medicament is negligible.
3. A new disc is used for every new operation.
4. Filtration is quite rapid.
5. They do not liberate particles or chemical substances to the filtrate.

Disadvantages

1. Fine pores may get clogged easily for which a prefilter may be used to remove colloidal matter.
2. Chemically they are less reistant and are soluble in certain organic solvents e.g. ketones and esters.
3. They are very brittle when dry and in this condition they can be stored for years together.

Membrane filters are extensively used for filtration and sterilization of a large number of pharmaceutical preparations such as parenteral preparations, ophthalmic solutions , biological preparations, hormones and enzymes. They are equally suitable for use in hospitals and in industries.

13.7 Maintaining Sterility Through Aseptic Techniques

Aseptic technique by itself is not a process of sterilization but is a procedure that does not allow the bacteria to introduce into the preparation from possible sources of contamination such as ingredients, solvents, mixing equipment, final containers, the working area and operator's hands and other contact parts.

Whenever any work is to be done aseptically , it must be performed in an area free from microorganisms known as aseptic area or in a room called aseptic room. The aseptic room has double door entry which are fitted with U.V. lamps. These lamps are also fitted above the working place. The operator should scrub his hands thoroughly with alcohol etc. and wear sterilized gloves, headgear, mask and clothings. All the apparatus and equipment required to be used in the process must be sterilized in advance.

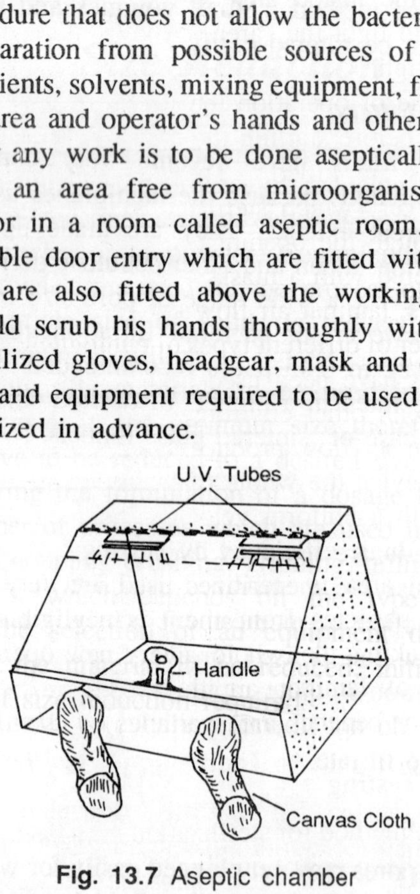

Fig. 13.7 Aseptic chamber

For small scale work, where aseptic rooms are not available i.e. for extemporaneous preparations, aseptic chamber is used. It is made up of wood over which sunmica can be fitted. In the front there are two openings each fitted with long piece of canvas cloth to prevent easy access of the microorganisms into the chamber. The upper slanting part is made of glass, upper half part of which is blackened so that U.V. rays may not fall directly on the eyes. This slanting glass is fixed with the top of the chamber by means of hinges. A handle is also provided to lift the slanting glass, when required. Inside top of the chamber is fitted with one or two ultra-violet tubes which makes the inside area sterile. A fluorescent tube is also provided to light the area. All the joints of the cabinet should be air tight.

At the time of operation the lights are switched on about 15-30 minutes before starting the experiment so that the inside microorganisms are killed. The hands thoroughly scrubbed with alcohol over which sterilized long gloves are worn are introduced through the openings of canvas cloth. The mouth should be covered with a mask.

Now a days, laminar air flow equipment is used for aseptic work. A number of different types of equipments for performing such operations have been used but laminar air flow devices are superior to all other environmental controls.

The laminar air flow produces a very clean and dust free area. In this device the whole of the air present in a confined area moves with a uniform velocity along parallel flow lines. By employing high efficiency bacteria proof filters, the air supplied to the area is sterilized which will sweep all dust and air borne particles from the chamber through the open side. Thus making the whole area free of microorganisms. Various types of laminar air flow devices in the form of room cabinets or benches are available.

13.8 Sterility Testing

Whatsoever method for sterilization may have been followed for sterilizing the preparations, each batch of pharmaceutical preparations required to be sterile must undergo sterility tests to confirm that they are free from microorganisms. It is not possible to perform sterility tests on each and every individual item, so, pharmacopoeias have prescribed that a specified amount of a drug or specified number of containers from a batch may be taken for testing.

Tests for sterility are based upon the principle that when a preparation containing bacteria is placed in a suitable medium which provide optimum conditions for bacterial growth e.g. nutrition, moisture, pH, presence or absence of air and incubate at a suitable temperature for sufficient time to allow the bacteria to grow, the presence of which will be indicated by the turbidity in the original medium. If there is no turbidity in the medium the preparation may be sterile.

Medium

Both, the aerobic and anaerobic media are required for sterility testing. For aerobic testing nutrient broth medium is used and for anaerobic testing thioglycolate medium is used.

Sampling

It is not possible that whole of the product or all the containers should be subjected to sterility testing only a suitable quantity from the bulk and desired number of containers from a "lot" may be taken for testing. A "lot" means that bulk of preparation or that group of containers which had been subjected to same sterilization procedures.

The pharmacopoeia states that from a 2 ml container or less, half of the quantity should be used for aerobic and other half for anaerobic testing. If the product is solid and weighs more than 100 mg than 50 mg for each test is used but if the quantity is less than 100mg then half the quantity should be used for each test. The liquid containers are selected at random and generally 2% or 20% containers, whichever is less, from a batch are subjected to sterility testing.

Procedure

According to U.S.P. there are two basic methods for sterility testing *(a) direct inoculation of test samples on culture media (b) filtration technique.*

In the direct inoculation method, an aliquot quantity of the material under test is transferred to culture tubes containing a measured volume of a suitable culture medium like fluid thiloglycolate medium or thioglycolate broth medium. This whole operation i.e. opening the containers taking aliquot quantity of the material under test and transferring it to the culture media contained in the tubes must be carried out under aseptic conditions and every precaution must be taken to prevent the accidental entry of microorganisms into the test. These tubes are plugged with sterile cotton wool and incubated for seven days at a temperature of 30 to 35°C. Positive and negative control tubes containing the culture media must be incubated under same conditions to confirm sterility and growth promoting properties of the medium . The material under test is considered sterile if there is no growth of microorganisms in the tubes but if there is any turbidity or growth then the test must be repeated 2nd time with fresh sample of material and culture medium because in the first test the bacterial growth may be due to accidental entry of microorganisms. If the 2nd test also shows growth, it may be repeated 3rd time very carefully and if this time also growth appears then the material fails to pass the sterility test.

If the product has antimicrobial properties they must be neutralized or eliminated by dilution. For solids or oily materials which make the culture medium turbid and make it difficult to conclude whether the turbidity is due to microbial growth or due to material itself, the normal test may have to be modified by subculturing the medium. If turbidity in substance does not appear the material is sterile but if turbidity appears it is due to microbial growth which shows that the material is not sterile.

13.9 Application of sterilization processes

The pharmacist uses sterilization process in pharmaceutical industries for sterilization of glassware and other equipments; for the preparation of injectables, ophthalmic, irrigating and other sterile dosage forms ; and for the dilution of sterile medicaments. However, it must be kept in mind that all types of medicaments and other articles cannot be sterilized by any one method, the pharmacist should have thorough knowledge of sterilization processes that for certain kind of medicament or article, whether dry heat, moist heat, filtration method or any other method is to be used.

In hospital practice the sterilization processes are used for the preparation of sterile gauzes and dressings; for sterilization of glass equipment like test tubes, petri dishes, pipettes, all glass syringes etc. for sterilization of operation theatre, and all types of articles used in operation theatre including aprons, gloves, face masks, hoods, forceps, scissors, knives etc.

The following articles/medicaments require sterilization:

(1) Glassware

The glassware and apparatus like flasks, beakers, funnels, dropper bottles, glass rods, pipettes, petridishes, glass tubes, pestle & mortar, tiles, ointment tubes, ampoules, vials , syringes, needles etc. may be sterilized either by moist heat or dry heat but dry heat method is preferred.

The glasswares should be thoroughly cleaned with soap and hot water to remove grease and then rinsed with apyrogenic water. New or very dirty articles should be soaked in cleansing solution overnight and then washed thoroughly. Then they are wrapped individually in brown paper or suitable grade of paper so that the external surfaces should remain uncontaminated. The apparatus is not unwapped until required for use. Flasks, beakers, tubes, pipettes etc. should be plugged with long fibre non-absorbent cotton wool.

The glassware so packed is kept on the shelves of the oven. Care must be taken that the articles are not tightly packed, there should be sufficient space in between the articles for the hot air to circulate. Contact with walls and floor of the oven must be prevented because these surfaces are more hot and may damage some of the articles and char cotton wool plugs and paper wrappings. The usual recommended minimum holding temperature and time for glassware is 180°C for 11 minutes.

When moist heat method is used it is essential that steam should come in contact with all the surfaces therefore a small quantity of water should be placed in the vessel otherwise they should be closed with a steam permeable closure. Sterilization is effected by heating at a temperature not lower than 160°C for one hour.

There are chances that the glassware may discolour and darken in colour if sterilized by ionizing radiations therefore not used.

(2) *Equipment*

Apparatus or devices made up of metal and surgical instruments, spatulas, metal part of bacterial filters such as millipore fitter, Seitz filter etc may be sterilized by steam under pressure at a temperature of 121°C for 15 to 30 minutes, depending on the size of instruments. The materials should be wrapped with muslin so that steam may penetrate to the surface of the metal parts.

Sharp edged instruments should not be sterilized in hot air because long heating at high temperatures in hot air lead to oxidation which reduces the sharpness of the blades.

(3) *Rubber and plastics*

Rubber articles such as stoppers, gloves, certain catheters and special feeding tubes may be sterilized in the autoclave at 121°C for 20 minutes; they must not be subjected to dry heat because high temperatures will spoil the rubber articles. Some synthetic rubbers such as silicon rubber has good heat resistance power therefore may be sterilized either by dry heat or moist heat.

Rubber teats, stoppers and closures should be made of high-quality materials which should release negligible amounts of undesirable substances and absorb minimum amount of solutions in contact with them. For sterilization they should be first boiled with 5 percent solution of sodium carbonate for 30-60 minutes to remove sulphur and other impurities present in rubber during manufacturing process. Then they are thoroughly washed with hot water, wrapped, sealed and sterilized in an autoclave at a temperature of 121°C for 20 minutes.

(4) *Aqueous/non-aqueous solutions and suspensions*

Thermostable aqueous solutions should be sterilized by steam under pressure in an autoclave at a temperature of 115°C to 118°C for 30 minutes but medicaments which are sufficiently thermostable may be sterilized at a temperature of 121°C for 15 minutes. Intravenous solutions such as dextrose and electrolytes; irrigating solution and all thermostable injections in ampoules or vials should be first clarified by filtration and then distributed to final containers under aseptic conditions which are then sealed and sterilized by steam under pressure.

Thermostable chemicals in solid state which get destroyed when they come in contact with moisture must be sterilized by dry heat. The substances which are sterilized in this way include powders such as zine oxide, kaolin, talc, starch, sulphonamides and surgical powders; fixed oils used as vehicles in oily injections; ophthalmic ointments, paraffins such as liquid paraffin, soft paraffin and hard paraffin; wool fat, wool alcohol, bees wax, glycerin etc. The powders or dry chemicals when sterilized by dry heat must be spread in thin layers so that adequate heat may penetrate. If the thickness of layers is large then exposure time must be increased. Unless otherwise stated in the monograph the substances must be exposed to dry heat in an oven at a temperature of 150°C for one hour or any other equally effective combination of time and temperature may be used.

Aqueous solutions of thermolabile drugs cannot be sterilized either by heating in an autoclave or heating with a bactericide. Such solutions or liquids may be sterilized by passing through bacteria proof filters under aseptic conditions. Asbestos filters should not be used where alternative filters are available because asbestos filters have tendency to shed fibres to the solution. As far as possible precautions should be taken to eliminate microorganisms at the time of preparation of solutions. Solutions sterilized by filtration are then transferred aseptically to previously sterilized final containers which are then sealed immediately so as to exclude microorganism. Pharmaceutical preparations which are sterilized by filtration include ophthalmic solutions, most ophthalmic alkaloidal solutions, antibiotic solutions and vitamin injections such as ascorbic acid etc.

(5) Surgical dressings and fabrics

The materials used in surgery and in the treatment of wounds and infections include cotton wool, gauze, gauze swabs, bandages, operation gowns, caps and masks, towels, trolly cloths and rubber sheets. These materials may be sterilized by dry heat, moist heat, ethylene oxide or ionising radiations.

Paraffin gauze dressings or dressings impregnated with soft paraffin may be sterilized by dry heat at a temperature not lower than 150°C for one hour. It must be ensured that all parts of the dressings come in contact with heat and they are maintained at this temperature for the stated time.

Surgical dressings made of cotton, rayon or other cellulose materials may be sterilized by moist heat. For this purpose the materials to be sterilized are loosely arranged in parallel layers in sterilizing chamber for satisfactory steam penetration and air removal. Precautions should be taken that the pack size must be as small as possible and heavy materials like towels and rubber sheets should, if possible, be sterilized reparately in small numbers apart from other materials.

For sterilization the air is removed from the chamber by reducing the pressure. Steam is then introduced until the required temperature is attained. This temperature is maintained for the appropriate period, after this the steam is removed from the chamber and drying is done by reducing the pressure in the chamber. Sterile air is then introduced through the filter, the chamber is opened and dressings are removed aseptically. Each container is labelled with date of sterilization to prevent long storage of the sterilized materials.

The materials which can withstand high temperatures may be exposed to 134°C for 3 minutes but most dressings and fabrics can be autoclaved at a temperature of 121°C to 122°C for 15 minutes.

13.10 Precautions for handling of sterilization equipment :

The aim of aseptic technique is to prevent contamination of materials, instruments, utensils, glass apparatus etc, during handling. The utensils and glass apparatus should be thoroughly washed with soap and water to remove dirt and grease then they are sterilized. After sterilization they should be removed from the oven/autoclave and stored under aseptic conditions for future use.

If possible aseptic work should be carried out in a separate room specially reserved for this purpose. In this room sterilized air (air which has been passed through bacteria proof filters) is introduced and a positive pressure is maintained so that the dust particles may not settle on the surface of the apparatus.

Likely sources of contamination include air, breath, hair, clothes, hands and the working surfaces. This contamination may be minimised:

(1) By introducing sterilized air under pressure into the working area.

(2) By wearing sterile/gowns, face masks and gloves.

(3) Hair should be covered with a sterilized cap and long hair should be tied at the back and covered.

(4) The skin should be thoroughly washed with soap and water and then any suitable antiseptic solution applied thereon.

(5) Before starting the aseptic work the working surfaces of table or bench should be scrubbed with a swab of disinfectant.

(6) Whenever strict aseptic conditions are required a number of bunsen burners may be lit around the working place. Preferably a gas lighter should be used for lighting the burners and paper ignited from another burner should never be used because it will scatter particles into the air.

(7) When transferring the sterilized equipment from one place to another a basket should be used so that only one journey is required and the room is not opened time and again.

14
Tablets

Tablets may be defined as the solid unit dosage form of medicament or medicaments with or without suitable diluents and prepared either by molding or by compression. They vary greatly in shape, size and weight which depends upon the amount of medicament and the mode of administration. Most commonly the tablets are disk shaped with covex surfaces but they are also available in special shapes like round, oval, oblong, cylindrical, square, triangular etc. They vary greatly in weight The tablets for oral administration may weigh from 0.2 to 0.8 gm including the diluents but the tablets meant for administration other than oral route may be lighter or heavier.

Tablets are the most widely used solid dosage form of medicament because they offer a number of advantages to the patient, prescriber, manufacturer and the manufacturing pharmacist. Because of these advantages their popularity is continuously increasing day by day.

Advantages

Tablets have following advantages:

1. They are easy to carry.
2. They are easy to swallow.
3. They are attractive in appearance.
4. Unpleasant taste can be masked by sugar coating.

5. They do no require any measurement of dose. The strip or blister packing has further facilitated the process of taking the dose by the patient. Moreover it provides a sealed covering which protects the tablets from atmospheric conditions like air, moisture and light etc.
6. Some of the tablets are divided into halves and quarters by drawing lines during manufacturing to facilitate breakage whenever a fractional dose is required.
7. An accurate amount of medicament even if very small can be incorporated.
8. Tablets provide prolonged stability to medicament.
9. The incompatibilities of medicaments and their deterioration due to environmental factors are less in tablet forms.
10. Since they are generally produced on a large scale therefore their cost of production is relatively low, hence economical.

14.1 Essential Qualities of a Good Tablet

1. They should be accurate and uniform in weight.
2. The drugs should be uniformly distributed throughout the tablets.
3. The size and shape should be reasonable for easy administration.
4. The tablets should not be too hard that it may not disintegrate in the stomach.
5. There should not be any incompatibilities.
6. They should be chemically and physically stable during storage.
7. They should not break during transportation or crumble in the hands of the patient.
8. They should be attractive in appearance.
9. There should not be any manufacturing defects like cracking, chipping or discoloration.
10. After administration it should disintegrate readily.
11. They should be easy and economical in production.

14.2 Types of Tablets

Mainly the tablets are classified into two classes (1) compressed tablets (2) molded tablets. The compressed tablets are usually prepared on large scale production methods whereas the molded tablets are prepared extemporaneously on a small scale. These two main types of tablets are further classified as follows:

Compressed Tablets

1. Oral tablets.
2. Chewable tablets.
3. Buccal/Sublingual tablets.
4. Lozenge tablets.
5. Soluble tablets.
6. Effervescent tablets.
7. Implants.
8. Vaginal tablets (Inserts).
9. Enteric coated tablets.
10. Sustained action tablets.
11. Sugar coated tablets.
12. Film coated tablets.
13. Layered tablets.
14. Press coated tablets.

Molded Tablets

1. Hypodermic tablets.
2. Dispensing tablets.

Molded Tablets or Tablet Triturates "TT"

Molded tablets are small disk shaped tablets which are prepared by forcing the soft mass into the cavities of the mold. Generally potent medicaments and highly toxic drugs in small doses are used for preparing the molded tablets. The potent medicament is diluted with a diluent like lactose, dextrose, sucrose or a mixture of lactose and sucrose. The mixed powders are moistened with a suitable dilution of alcohol (generally 50% alcohol is used) and mixed thoroughly so as to get a soft mass. The soft mass so prepared is pressed into the perforations of the mold with a spatula. The excess of the mass is removed by applying pressure over the spatula. This perforated plate of the mold filled with the mass is placed over another plate having exactly the same number of projecting pegs as that of perforations and these projecting pegs completely fit into the holes. A little pressure is applied over top plate which will force the plate move downward, leaving the molded tablets on the projecting pegs. The ejected tablets are spread in single layers on clean surface and dried either by keeping in a warm place or hot air oven.

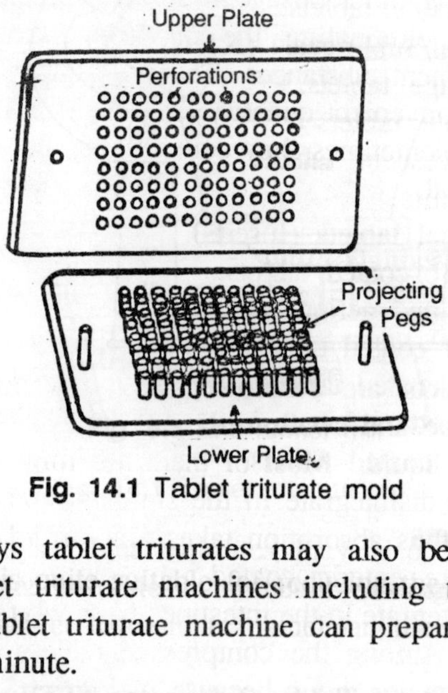

Fig. 14.1 Tablet triturate mold

Now a days tablet triturates may also be prepared on automatic tablet triturate machines including tablet making machines. A tablet triturate machine can prepare 2500 tablet triturates per minute.

Hypodermic tablets

Hypodermic tablets are soft readily soluble tablets which are made in a tablet triturate mould. They are used for preparing solutions to be injected, therefore in selecting the materials used for preparing the hypodermic tablets care must be taken that they should be completely and readily soluble and no insoluble particle should be present. They should be free from bacterial contamination and proper precautions should be taken during molding regarding contamination and cleanliness.

Since the solutions prepared from hypodermic tablets are rarely sterile and a number of sterile parenteral solutions are now available therefore the use of hypodermic tablets for preparing solution for injections is being discouraged.

Dispensing Tablets

These tablets are prepared for providing an accurate and convenient quantity of a drug that can be incorporated readily in compounding other dosage forms e.g. liquids, powders, or capsules thus eliminating the necessity of weighing small quantities of potent substances. These tablets are solely designed to provide a convenient quantity for administration as a dosage form because sometimes they contain very potent drugs which may prove fatal.

Compressed Tablets

1. Oral Tablets

These tablets are swallowed as such. They are placed over the tongue and swallowed with a drink of water or any other suitable liquid. Most of them are formulated in such a way that they disintegrate in the stomach and dissolve in the gastric fluids thus absorption takes place from there. Some of the tablets like enteric coated tablets pass the stomach as such and disintegrate in the intestines from where the absorption takes place. Among the compressed tablets the oral tablets constitute the major group because majority of the compressed tablets are meant for oral administration.

Since the oral tablets are required to be disintegrated in a very short time therefore either the medicaments itself should be freely soluble in gastro-intestinal fluids or disintegrating agent must be added in the formulation of tablets.

2. Chewable Tablets

These are the tablets which are required to be broken and chewed in between the teeth before ingestion. These tablets are given to the children who have difficulty in swallowing and to the adults who dislike swallowing. A number of antacid tablets and multivitamin tablets are prepared as chewable tablets.

For the preparation of chewable tablets mannitol is used as a base. It is a white crystalline, chemically inert, nonhygroscopic, thermostable powder and is as sweet as that of glucose. It does not have any objectionable effects but since it is expensive so it cannot be used in tablets of low cost, therefore other substances like sorbitol lactose, chocolate powder, dextrose and glycine can be substituted in place of mannitol.

These tablets should have very acceptable taste and flavour. They should disintegrate in a short time and produce cool sweet taste. Chewable tablets can be taken at any place even if water is not available. These tablets do not require any disintegrating agent to be present in the formulation. The use of gums and other substances which produce hard granules should be avoided. The lubricants used should have agreeable taste.

3. *Buccal/Sublingual Tablets*

These tablets are required to be placed below the tongue (sublingual) or in the side of the cheek (buccal) for the slow release of the medicament except in the case of nitroglycerin and mannitol hexanitrate tablets which should dissolve in 1 to 2 minutes to produce immediate effect.

Generally these types of tablets contain those drugs which are destroyed, inactivated or not absorbed in the G.I.T. but are directly absorbed through the mucosal tissues of the oral cavity. These tablets contain large proportions of sweetening agents like mannitol and/or sucrose to impart sweetness.

4. *Lozenge Tablets*

These tablets should not disintegrate in the oral cavity but should dissolve slowly in the mouth to produce continuous effect on the mucous membrane of the throat. They can be prepared by molding as well as by compression method. The lozenges prepared by compression are known as lozenge tablets,

In the formulation of lozenges no disintegrating agent is included rather the quantity of binding agent is increased so as to produce slow dissolution. The formulation must contain sweetening and flavoring agents.

5. Soluble Tablets

These tablets are required to dissolve completely in the liquid to produce solution of definite concentration. The solutions prepared by dissolving the soluble tablets may include mouth washes, gargles, skin lotions, douches, antibiotics and certain vitamins. The use of soluble tablets, 'hypodermic tablets' for the preparation of injectable solutions is restricted because the solutions so prepared are not sterile.

For the preparation of soluble tablets all the ingredients used in the formulation must be completely soluble in solvent.

6. Effervescent Tablets

These tablets alongwith the active medicament contain other ingredients like sodium bicarbonate, citric acid and tartaric acid which react in the presence of water liberating carbon dioxide and producing effervescence leading to disintegration of the tablet, thus hastens solution formation and increases the palatability. These tablets have the advantage over effervescent powders of being in tablet dosage form.

7. Vaginal Tablets (Inserts)

Sometimes vaginal suppositories or pessaries are prepared by compression which are known as vaginal tablets. Antibiotics and steroids are formulated in this way. Soluble additives are used for their preparation. They are generally ovoid or almond shaped for ease of insertion. Plastic tube inserters can also be used for placing these tablets in vaginal tract.

Some laxative suppositories are also formulated as compressed tablets. The active medicaments are mixed with such disintegrating agents which either swell up after absorbing moisture or produce effervescence thus facilitating disintegration. These rectal tablets are covered with thin layers of polyethylene glycol which act as protective covering and also facilitate the insertion of these tablets into the rectum.

8. Implants

Implants are small tablets meant for insertion under the skin by giving as small surgical cut into the skin which is stitched after the insertion of the tablet. Since these tablets are to be implanted intramuscularly or subcutaneously therefore they must be sterile. They must be prepared under aseptic conditions and packed in unit dose sterile containers.

Implants are prepared to provide a slow and continuous release of the drug over prolonged periods of time ranging from 3 months to 6 months or even more. Due to this reason the drugs used in the preparation of implants are water insoluble, no excipients are used and they are compressed under heavy pressure. These tablets are more commonly used in veterinary medicine than human medicine. They can also be used for birth control in human beings. Generally steroidal hormones like testosterone, stilbesterol etc. are formulated as implants.

9. Enteric Coated Tablets

These are the tablets which are required to be disintegrated in the intestines and not in the stomach. They are given coating which makes the tablet to pass the stomach as such but breaks in the alkaline medium of the intestines.

10. Sustained Action Tablets

These are the tablets which after oral administration release the drug at a desired time and prolong the effect of the medicament. Repeat action tablets are used to periodically release a complete dose of the drug to the G.I.T. fluids thus maintaining a constant blood concentration.

11. Sugar Coated Tablets

These are the compressed tablets which are given a sugar coating to mask the objectionable taste and odour of the drug as well as to protect the substances from atmospheric conditions. To make elegant they can be given suitable colour coating.

12. Film Coated Tablets

These are the compressed tablets which are given a thin coating of water soluble materials which protect the drug substances from atmospheric conditions. Various polymers are used for film coating.

13. Layered Tablets

These are the compressed tablets in which the granules of incompatible substances are compressed into two or more layers successively in the same tablet. Special tablet making machines are required for making layered tablets.

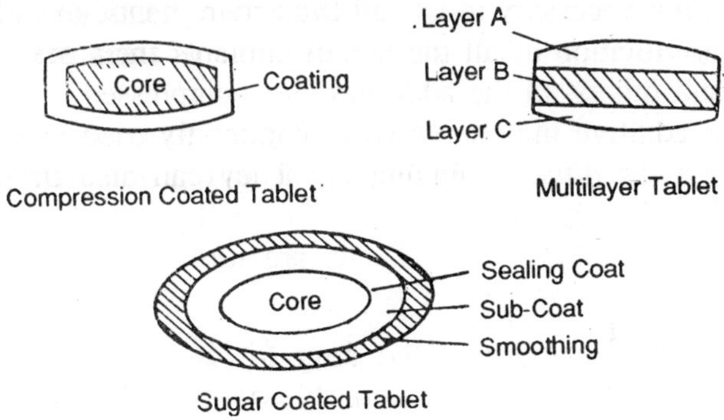

Fig. 14.2 Different types of tablets

14. Press Coated Tablets

In press coated tablets the granules of incompatible ingredients are compressed around the previously compressed tablet. These type of tablets are made on special tablet making machines in two successive compressions. These types of tablets can also be used for giving enteric coating and sustained release to the medicaments.

14.3 Formulation of tablets

Compressed tablets usually consists of active medicaments mixed with a number of inert substances known as excipients or additives. These additives are added to give the qualities of a good tablet. Although these additives are termed as inert but they have a great influence on stability, bioavailability and the process by which the dosage forms are prepared. According to the functions which these additives play in the preparation of tablets may be classified as follows:

1. Diluents.
2. Binders.
3. Granulation agents.
4. Disintegrating agents.
5. Lubricants.
6. Colouring agents.
7. Flavouring agents.
8. Sweetening agents.

It is not necessary to use all the above mentioned additives in the formulation of all the tablets some of them may require a few and others all the additives.

One additive may serve two or more functions e.g. starch may serve as diluent, binding agent and disintegration agent in one form or the other.

1. Diluents

When the quantity of the drug for an individual dose is very small and it is not practicable to compress such small amount in the form of a tablet then the inert substances which are added to increase the bulk of powders to be easily compressed are known as diluents. Various diluents used are: lactose, sodium chloride, starch, powdered sucrose, mannitol, calcium carbonate, calcium sulphate, calcium phosphate etc.

2. Binders

Some substances which are available in the crystalline form can be compressed directly but majority of the drugs will have to be converted to granules before compression. The agents used during granulation to impart cohesiveness to the powdered substances are known as binders. They keep the tablet intact after compression. Various commonly used binders are: starch, acacia, tragacanth, gelatin, glucose, lactose, sucrose, methyl cellulose etc.

In some formulations binders are used in the dry form whereas in others they are used as liquids by dissolving them in a suitable solvent like water, alcohol or a mixture of these two. The proportion of binding agents has to vary from product to product. The tablets which are required to keep intact for a long time like lozenges and implants need high percentage of binders whereas tablets which should disintegrate in a short time need low proportion of binders.

3. Granulating Agents

Granulating agents are the substances which are added to powders during granulating process to convert fine powders into granules. The quantity of proper granulating agent to be incorporated is very critical. Insufficient quantity of granulating agent may lead to poor adhesion, soft tablets and 'capping', whereas excessive quantity may lead to hard tablets with greater disintegration time. In addition the wet screening may be more difficult if excessive granulating agent is present. The commonly used granulating agents are: water, mucilages of acacia, tragacanth and starch; liquid glucose, syrup and alcohol in various dilutions.

4. Disintegrating Agents

Disintegrating agents or disintegrators are the substances or a mixture of substances which are added to tablets to facilitate their disintegration or breaking apart into small particles in G.I.T. after administration, thus facilitating dissolution. Generally two types of disintegrating agents are used (i) substances which swell up when they come in contact with moisture (ii) substances which react with effervescence when they come in contact with moisture.

The most popular and commonly used disintegrating agents of first type are maize starch and potato starch. These starches have great affinity for water and swell up when they come in contact with water thus breaking the tablet apart. The other disintegrating agents include veegum, methyl cellulose, agar, bentonite, carboxy methyl cellulose and citrus pulp. Some manufacturers use sodium lauryl sulphate alongwith starch as disintegrating agent. This produces better wetting of the granules resulting in faster dissolution rate of drugs.

The second type of disintegrating agents include a combination of sodium bicarbonate, citric acid and tartaric acid. When this combination comes in contact with moisture present in the stomach produces effervescence thus disintegrating the tablet.

Generally disintegrating agents are added in two portions. The major part is incorporated to the powders before granulation and the other mixed with the dried granules alongwith lubricants. Disintegrants added in this manner serve two purposes. The disintegrant added after granulation breaks the tablet apart into granules and the portion added before granulation breaks the granules into fine particles thus facilitating the dissolution of drugs. The disintegration time of a tablet depends upon many factors e.g. quantities of diluents, binders, lubricants, tablet hardness, size of granules and coatings.

5. Lubricants

Lubricants are the substances which are added to granules before compression to improve the flow of granules from the hopper to the die cavity by reducing interparticle friction, to prevent adhesion of the powders to the surface of dies and punches thus reducing wear and tear of dies and punches and to facilitate the ejection of the tablet from the die cavity after compression. Commonly used lubricants are: magnesium stearate, calcium stearate, stearic acid, and talc. Other materials such as cocoa butter, hydrogenated vegetable oils, liquid paraffin, hard paraffin, waxes and wax like materials may also be used as lubricants to prevent adhesiveness to the surface of dies and punches.

6. Colouring Agents

Colouring agents are used to impart elegance to the tablets. Sometimes they are also used to identify the different types of tablets. Only the approved colours are used. These colours may be added either in the mixed powders before granulation or they may be dissolved in the vehicles used for making the granules. The latter procedure gives more uniform colour.

7. Flavouring Agents

Generally flavours are added to all lozenges, chewable tablets and effervescence tablets. Voltaile oils, volatile substances and fruit flavours are used for this purpose. The volatile substances are dissolved in a suitable organic solvent and sprayed over the granules before compression. Fruit flavours and spray dried beadlets are incorporated to the mixed powders before granulation.

8. Sweetening Agents

Sweetening agents are added to the tablets which are required to be dissolved in the buccal cavity. The bases for their formulation are already sweet e.g. mannitol, lactose and sucrose. They impart sweetness of varying degree. The additional sweetness may be imparted by including additional quantity of sucrose and artificial sweetening agents like cyclamates and saccharin. But the use of cyclamates and saccharin have already been banned therefore sugars can be included to impart an acceptable taste.

14.4 Preparation of Tablets

In the preparation of tablets the fine powders are not used but they are prepared in the form of granules which are then compressed. The granules so prepared have certain advantages over fine powders in that:

(i) The granules flow evenly through the hopper resulting in tablets of uniform weight whereas the fine powders does not flow evenly through the hopper which produces tablets of varying weights.

(ii) The drugs are uniformly mixed and bound together in the form of granules thereby the mixed drugs do not separate out whereas in a powder containing several ingredients; the vibrations of the machine separates the materials, the heavy materials move downwards thereby the resulting tablets may not be uniform in composition.

(iii) The very fine powders have a tendency to blow out of the die and stick to the sides of the punches. Granules being heavier do not have this difficulty.

Proper size of the granules must be prepared. No.12 to No. 20 mesh size granules are considered most suitable. It is not necessary that the whole material must be in granules, usually a small proportion 10 to 20% of fine powder must also be present which produces smoother tablets. Large size granules are not preferred because they may not feed into the dies as evenly or compress well as those of granules of proper size.

14.5 Methods of Preparation of Tablets

There are three methods by which compressed tablets can be prepared.

1. Direct Compression.
2. Dry Granulation.
3. Wet Granulation.

1. Direct Compression

The materials which are available in crystalline form and have free flowing and binding characteristics can be compressed directly, but the majority of the drugs cannot be compressed easily in this way because sometimes they produce tablets which may not disintegrate. To overcome this difficulty directly compressible vehicles can be incorporated to the drug and compressed. Such vehicles include spray dried lactose, anhydrous lactose, calcium phosphate, compressible sugar, mannitol and microcrystaline cellulose. The drugs which can be compressed directly are: sodium chloride, sodium bromide, sodium salicylate, potassium chloride, potassium bromide, potassium iodide, potassium nitrate, ammonium chloride, acetyl salicylic acid crystals, potassium permanganate and methenamine etc. These materials possess necessary cohesive and flow properties thereby they can be easily compressed.

2. Dry Granulation

This method is also known as slugging, precompression or double compression method. In this method the blend of powders are compressed into slugs on specially designed tablet machines. The slugs are the flat faced large size tablets which are prepared under heavy pressure on tablet press. These slugs are then broken to suitable size granules by passing through an oscillating granulator or other suitable device fitted with No.10 or No.20 sieve. The resultant granules are mixed with lubricants and other necessary additives, then they are compressed into finished tablets in the usual way.

3. Wet Granulation

This is the most widely and general method used in the preparation of tablets. This method is popular because the granulation meets all the qualities required for a good tablet but has the disadvantage that materials which are destroyed by moisture or excessive heat cannot be prepared by wet granulation. Moreover this method is time consuming and requires a number of persons as many different steps are involved in the preparation. The steps involved are weighing, mixing, granulation, sieving the wet mass, drying, sieving the dried mass, lubrication and compression.

In this method the crystalline substances are reduced to fine powder, they are mixed with other ingredients, major portion of the disintegrating agent is incorporated and mixed uniformly. The mixed powders thus obtained are passed through a sieve No. 30 to 60. Dry binding agent if any added followed by the careful addition of granulating agent or binding solution. The addition of proper quantity of granulating agent is very important because if the quantity is less this will lead to poor adhesion, soft tablets and capping whereas the excessive quantity of binding agent will lead to the formation of a very hard tablet which will take a longer disintegrating time. It may also be more difficult to pass the excessive wet mass through the sieves to get proper granules. A rough method to determine the proper quantity of granulating agent to be added can be determined by pressing a portion of the mass in the palm of the hand, if the ball breaks under moderate pressure, the mixture is ready for screening. After adding the proper quantity of the granulating agent to the powders they are mixed continuously until uniform mass is obtained. The wet mass so obtained is then passed through sieve No. 6 to 20. On large scale manufacturing various types of granulating machines can be used. The wet granules obtained after passing through the various sieves are spread in thin layers in trays and dried in an oven at a temperature not exceeding 60°C. The dried granules are broken up and passed through a proper screen to obtain the granules of proper size. The granules are then mixed with other additives like the second portion of disintegrants, lubricants and flavouring agents etc. The blended granules are thus ready for compression.

Out of the above mentioned method of preparation of tablets, the slugging or dry granulation method is considered more suitable because the possible reactions due to heat and moisture are avoided. Moreover the tablets prepared from dry granulation method are more uniform in composition and disintegrate more rapidly than tablets made by other methods. This method also involves lower cost of equipment, labour and handling. Due to the above mentioned advantages the dry granulation method is becoming more popular and being widely used in the pharmaceutical industry.

14.6 Tablet Compression

For the compression of granules in the form of tablets, various types of machines are used which are known as tablet making machines or tablet presses. Various types of machines so used are as follows:

1. Single punch machines.
2. Multi punch machines.
3. Rotary tablet machines.
4. High-speed rotary tablet machines.
5. Multilayer rotary tablet machines.

1. Single Punch Machines

In these types of machines one set of die and punch is fitted and only one tablet can be compressed at one time. They are used when small quantity of tablets are to be prepared.

They may be hand operated or power operated and with these machines 60 to 90 tablets per minute can be prepared.

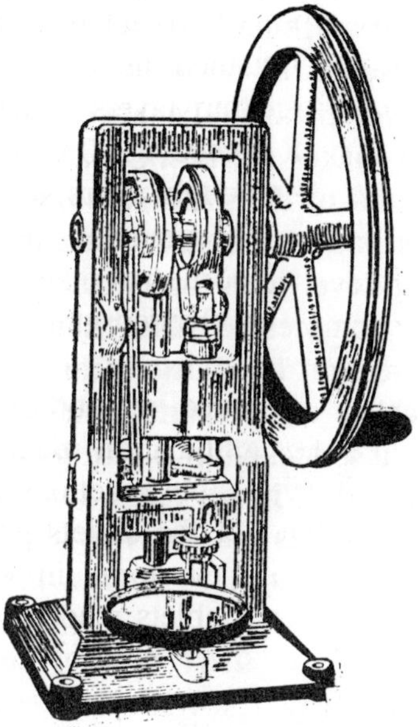

Fig. 14.3 Hand operated single punch tablet making machine

Single punch, hand operated or power operated tablet making machines are made up of good quality of steel frame with heavy base. The horizontal plate of the frame is fitted with a die which is held firmly in place by means of a screw. The vertical shaft holds a lower punch which moves freely in the die. On the lower side of the shaft, capacity regulating screw and ejection regulating screws are fitted by which the volume and weight of the granules to be compressed and ejection of the tablet after compression can be adjusted. The upper punch having the same diameter as that of lower punch is fixed and locked into its holder in the upper part of the shaft. The pressure to be applied is also adjusted from here. The upper punch enters the die correctly on its downward movement. A hopper shoe is provided in which the granules to be compressed are filled. A driving wheel is attached to the shaft which may be hand operated or driven by a motor. The parts of a hand operated tablet making machine are shown in the diagram.

Working

The granulated material ready for compression is placed in the hopper of the machine from where it feeds into the die, where it is compressed in between two punches, the upper punch and the lower punch. The lower punch is adjusted in such a way that it makes sufficient space in the die cavity to hold weighed amount of the material so as to make the tablet of required weight and at the same time the top of the lower punch should be in level with the upper surface of the die for easy ejection of the compressed tablet from the die. The pressure required for compression is adjusted from the upper punch. A number of trial tablets are prepared and when the machine is adjusted correctly, it is locked in position and required number of tablets are prepared. When a large number of tablets are to be prepared, the materials can be put into the large feeding cup attached to the hopper. This avoids, the frequent refilling of the hopper.

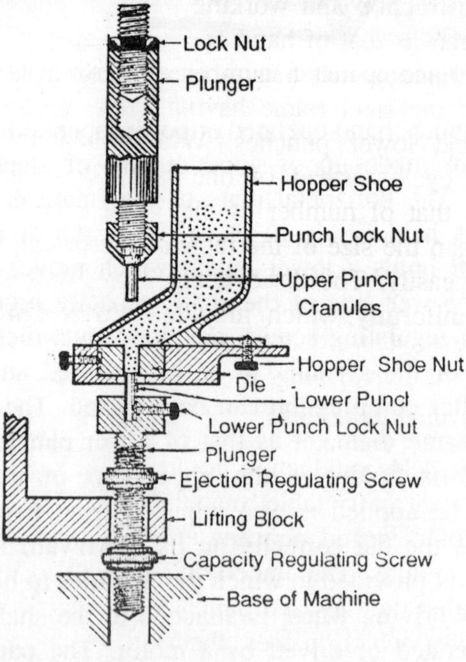

Fig. 14.4 Hand operated single punch tablet making machine showing different parts

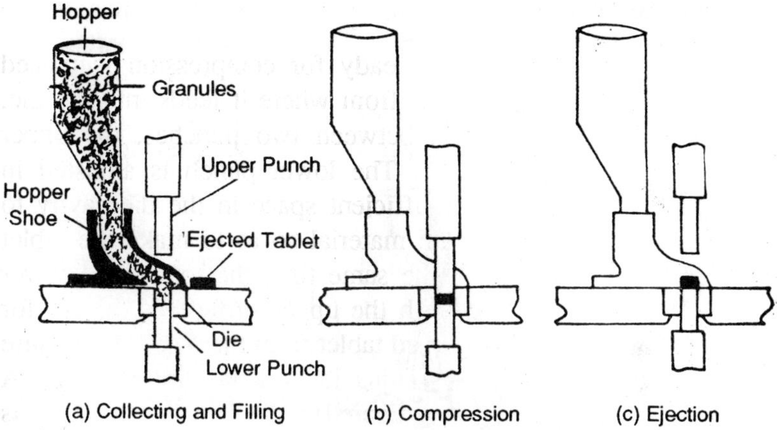

Fig. 14.5 Hand operated single punch tablet making machine showing compression cycle

2. Multi Punch Machines

The construction and working of multi punch machines is exactly similar as that of hand operated single punch machines with the difference that a number of dies varying from 2-12 are fitted in the steel frame having exactly the same number of upper and lower punches. With multi punch machines, during one cycle instead of one tablet as many tablets are prepared as that of number of dies. These types of machines are used when the size of the tablets is small and pressure can be adjusted easily. The disadvantages are that all the dies are not filled uniformly which may lead to weight variation in tablets.

3. Rotary Tablet Machines

For large scale production, rotary tablet machines are used. The high speed rotary tablet machines are fitted with as many as 70 sets of dies and punches and can produce upto 10000 tablets per minute. The underlying principle of rotary tablet machine is that the dies and punches are mounted in a rotating holder (turret) which passes them in sequence through the filling, compression and ejection stages at a much faster speed whereby the output is increased to a great extent.

The essential features of the rotary machine is that it has a circular rotating head which is divided into three parts:

(a) an upper part which carries the upper punches
(b) a central part which carries the dies.
(c) a lower part which carries the lower punches.

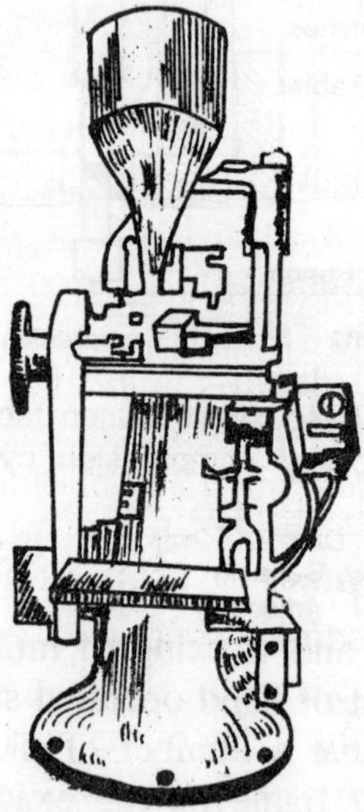

Fig. 14.6 Rotary tablet machine

All these parts are arranged in a circle around the rotating head. A large hopper is fitted which supplies the granules to the 'feed frame' placed over the central part containing the dies. As the head rotates, the dies come one by one under the feed frame and are filled. The upper and lower punches passing in between rollers, gradually compress the granules in the form of tablets which are pushed out.

4. Multilayer Rotary Tablet Machines

With multilayer rotary tablet machines, tablets having one, two or three layers can be produced. They have the advantage that incompatible drugs can be compressed in different layers and separating these layers with an inert material. Sustained action preparations can also be prepared by this method.

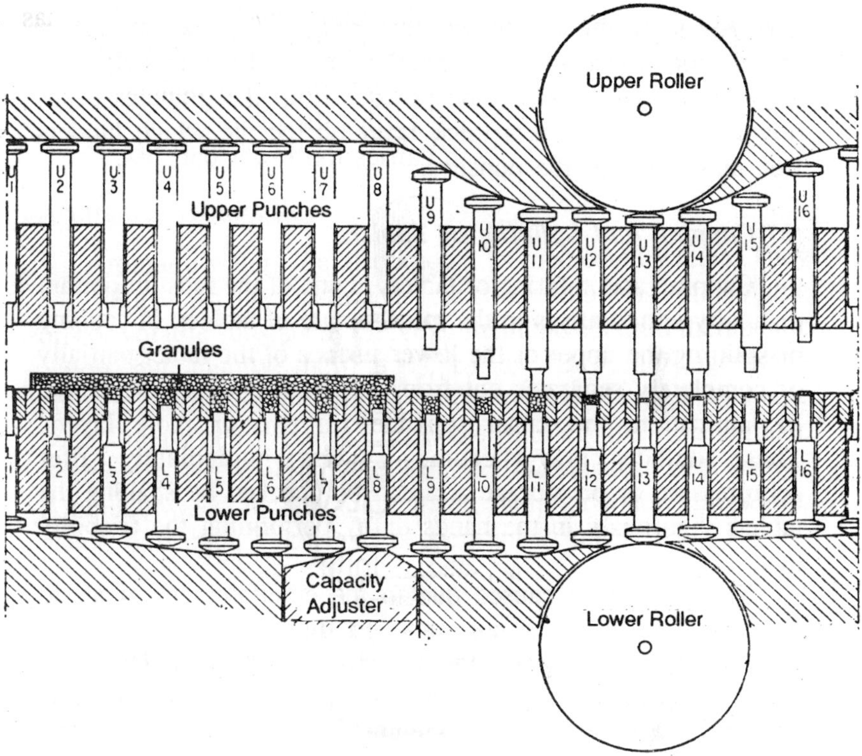

Fig. 14.7 Rotary tablet machine showing the compression cycle

14.7 Manufacturing Defects in Tablets

During the routine production of tablets so many defects arise with the finished tablets which may be due to either some faults in the formulation or in the tableting equipment and sometimes due to both of these reasons. Some defects are noticed immediately during manufacturing but others may be noticed on storage as in the case of capping. Therefore it is important to perform tests at the start and during production in order to take prompt remedial action. These defects are described below:

(a) Binding in the Die

During binding in the die the ejection of the tablet is difficult and is often accompanied by a characteristic noise.

The edges of the tablets become rough. This defect occurs due to poor lubrication of granules, under dried granules and dirty or worn out dies. Fine powder from the granules seeps downwards and forms a thick layer on the die which hinders free movement of the punches.

(b) Capping and Splitting of Tablets

Capping and splitting of tablets is one of the most important difficulty which arises in the manufacture of tablets. In capping or splitting the upper or the lower surface of the tablet partially or completely separates out from the main body of the tablet. In lamination, the tablet separates in two or more layers. These defects may become evident immediately after compression or on storage and can be checked by shaking the tablets vigorously in the hands or by performing the friability test.

The capping is caused due to the entertainment of air in the granules which is not removed during compression but escapes afterwards when the pressure is released. This may also be caused due to the presence of either excess of fine powder in granules or less amount of fines in granules. The use of too soft granules also leads to capping. The wear and tear of punches and dies is also responsible for capping. The wrong setting of dies and punches is another reason of capping.

These types of difficulties can be corrected by regranulating the material, altering the pressure adjustments or reducing the speed of the machine. The worn out dies and punches must be replaced and the level of the top of the lower punch must be corrected so as to coincide with the level of the upper surface of the die. Proper granules and required amount of fine powders must be used to avoid capping.

(c) Picking and Sticking

These are two synonymous terms and can be used one for the other. In picking a small surface of the tablet material is removed by the punches and adheres to the surface of punches, therefore the resulting tablets show a pitted surface instead of smooth surface. This may be caused due to the presence of scratches on the punches or by using wet granules during compression. In sticking, the granules adhere to the die wall and thereby the lower punch cannot move freely. This trouble may be due to the use of damp granules or due to worn out dies and punches. These defects can be removed by using the dry granules and by adding a lubricant to the granules. The worn out dies and punches must be replaced. The use of chromium plated punches also overcomes this difficulty and produces tablets with smooth surface.

(d) Mottling

This defect occurs in the coloured tablets. The colour does not distribute evenly throughout the tablet, zones of different shades appear on the surface of the tablet. This defect may be caused either due to the difference of colours in the drugs and the added excipients or due to the migration of dyes during drying of granules. This defect can be overcome by using a dye which can mask the colours of tablet ingredients, by changing the solvent system or by drying the granules at a low temperature.

(e) Weight Variation

Excessive weight variation occurs between tablets during manufacture. This problem is due to the following reasons:

(i) Poor flow of granules to the die.
(ii) Size separation of granules i.e. small and large size granules.
(iii) Presence of too fines in the granules.
(iv) Separation of the mixed ingredients of granules.
(v) Less quantity or poor mixing of lubricants.
(vi) Due to automatic change in the adjustment of punches.
(vii) In rotary tablet making machines this defect is due to unequal length of lower punches.

(f) Hardness Variation

The tablets vary greatly in hardness. The reasons for this variation are the same as discussed under weight variation. Apart from these reasons other factors include weight of material, space between the upper and lower punches at the time of compression, pressure applied on the upper punches and excessive proportions of fatty lubricant such as magnesium stearate. The hardness may also increase on normal storage of tablets. Therefore it is important to note that the tablets should not be harder than required. The hard tablets may not disintegrate in the required period of time and too soft tablets may not withstand the hazards during handling, transporting and dispensing.

(g) Double Impression

This defect occurs in those tablets on which letters are printed. This involves only lower punch which have a monogram the impression of which is printed on the tablet during compression. On some machines the punch moves downwards and then travel uncontrolled upward to a short distance to push the tablet out of the die. During its free travel it rotates and makes second impression on the tablet. This impression is generally lighter than the original impression. The new tablet making machines are fitted with devices which prevents the rotation of the lower punch.

14.8 Tablet Coating

Tablets were originally coated for the sake of pharmaceutical elegance by improving their appearance, taste and stability. More recently coating has been used to control the site of drug release (enteric coating) and delay or prolong the release of drug from the dosage form (sustained action) and hence the absorption of drug or drugs present. The nature of coating varies, it may be simple or complex. In its simplest form it may merely consist of a thin film of varnish, applied to make the tablets dust free and reduce any bitter taste. In most complex form it may consist of inner and outer shell enclosing different types of drugs which may be incompatible or are required to be released at a specified time.

14.9 Sugar Coating

The most important is sugar coating of tablets. It is one of the oldest and most commonly used method of coating the tablets on a commercial scale. It is used to mask the unpleasant taste and odour, to improve the appearance and to protect the ingredients from decompensation on exposure to air and moisture.

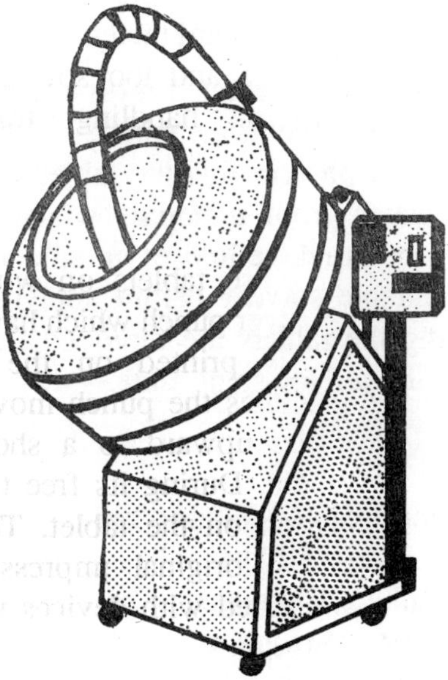

Fig. 14.8 Tablet coating pan

Tablets which are to be coated are made with convex surfaces instead of flat surfaces because the tablets with convex surfaces are easier to coat than with flat surfaces. The compressed tablets are shaken on sieves to remove any fine powder and broken tablets before placing them in the coating pan. The coating pans are spherical vessels made of copper or stainless steel which rotate on the axis driven by a motor. The polishing pans consist of canvas drums which may be rotated on the same machine after removing the coating pan. The pans are fitted with air blowers to force hot or cold air to facilitate drying. They are also fitted with exhaust pipes to remove the unwanted dusting powders and moisture from the coating pans.

The various stages involved in sugar coating are:

1. Water proofing.
2. Subcoating.

3. Smoothing.
4. Colouring and finishing.
5. Polishing.

1. Water Proofing

Since water is used as a vehicle for dissolving sugar required for coating, when it will come in contact with the drugs they may be destroyed. To prevent this the tablets are given one or two coatings of water proof materials which may consist of arsenic free shellac, ethyl cellulose or silicones. They must be dissolved in suitable solvent before applying. After giving water proof coating the tablets are removed from the pan and allowed to dry in the air for some time.

2. Sub-Coating

The water proof coated tablets are put in the pan and rotated. On the rotating tablets a heavy syrup consisting of acacia and sugar solution is added. The tablets are allowed to roll until they become sticky and adhere to each other and to the pan. At this point the tablets are dusted with dusting powder which may consist of talc, starch, powdered acacia or precipitated chalk until they lose their tendency to adhere to each other. Rotation of the pan is continued until the tablets are fully dried. Subsequent coatings are applied by using alternatively syrup and dusting powder until the edges of tablets are sufficiently covered and rounded. Care should be taken that before giving the next coating the first one must have been thoroughly dried. At this stage the subcoated tablets are removed from the pan and allowed to dry. The pan is washed to carry out the next stage.

3. Smoothing

The subcoated tablets are put in the pan and rotated. They are given a few coatings of heavy sugar syrup which are dried simultaneously until a smooth surface is obtained and tablets of specific size are produced. The tablets are removed and pan washed.

4. *Colouring*

For colouring the tablets, the desired water soluble colour is dissolved in the diluted syrup. Several coatings of this coloured diluted syrup are given, drying each time. Then few coatings of undiluted coloured syrup are given. Drying should be carried out after each addition but the last coating must be dried at a very slow speed to prevent sticking of the tablets with each other and to dry the tablets at a slow rate.

5. *Polishing*

For polishing, the thoroughly dried coated tablets are transferred to canvas drum known as polishing pan. The polishing pan is rotated and lumps of wax or solution of wax dissolved in some volatile solvent is added. The tablets are allowed to rotate until the volatile solvent evaporates and a desired finish is obtained.

14.10 Film Coating

A more recent method of coating the tablets is film coating. Although the film coated tablets are possibly less elegant in appearance but they are considered more satisfactory than sugar coated tablets because in film coating various steps like water proofing, subcoating and smoothing are unnecessary thereby the coating time is reduced to a great extent, ultimately the cost of production is decreased and tablets of better strength are produced.

The coating materials such as sodium carboxy methyl cellulose and other cellulosic high polymers have been used to mask the unpleasant taste and odour. Polyethylene glycol and carbowax 6000 can also be used as coating materials. These materials are dissolved in a volatile solvent and added or sprayed to the tablets rotating in a coating pan. If the tablets are to be coloured, the dyes are dissolved in the solvent and sprayed over the tumbling tablets. The tablets are allowed to dry so as to form a permanent film over the tablets.

14.11 Compression Coating

This method is also known as press coating or dry coating as no water or any solvent is used in the coating. Only the dried granules are compressed around the precompressed tablets. This method is applicable to those drugs which are decomposed in the presence of moisture. Incompatible materials can be incorporated by pressing them in different coatings. One material can be compressed on the core and still another can be compressed on the core and the first coating. Similarly repeat action tablets can be prepared by coating the tablets with an appropriate material.

The process of compression coating is applied by compressing the granules in the form of a core tablet. The core so formed is fed to the die of another press to which the granules of the material to be coated are already supplied. The tablet is then compressed between the punches of the press. Similarly the second coat can be applied by supplying the coated tablet to the third press and compressed there along with the granules meant for second coating.

14.12 Enteric Coating

Enteric coating is applied to the tablets which are required to pass the stomach as such but readily disintegrate in the intestines. The substances which are generally given enteric coating are those: (a) which are decomposed in the acidic medium of the stomach (b) which produce irritation in the stomach (c) the action of which is required only in the intestines (d) absorption of which takes place from the intestines (e) delayed action of which is required.

The commercially used materials for enteric coating include fats and fatty acids, shellac and shellac derivatives and the cellulose acetate phthalates. Now-a-days the products so produced are generally coated with cellulose acetate phthalates because they give most satisfactory enteric coatings.

An alcoholic solution of arsenic free shellac may be sprayed on the tablets rotating in a coating pan. Tablets are allowed to rotate until the alcohol evaporates and tablets dried by means of a current of hot air. Cellulose acetate phthalate is dissolved in an organic solvent like ethyl acetate or alcohol and sprayed over the tablets rotating in the coating pan. Solvent is allowed to evaporate and tablets dried by means of hot air.

The cellulose acetate phthalate coated tablets must be sealed with coating of wax to prevent penetration of water. A plasticizer can also be used to reduce the cracks in the films.

14.13 Microencapsulation

Microencapsulation is placed in the section of capsules only because of the relationship in terminology to that of encapsulation. Since the drugs are given coatings therefore it is discussed under coating procedures.

Microencapsulation is a process or technique by which solids, liquids or dispersions are given thin coatings of microscopic size ranging from several tenths of a micron to 5000 μ in size.

In literature there are a number of methods available for microencapsulation which include air suspension, coacervation-phase separation, electrostatic deposition, spray drying and congealing; and pan coating techniques but here coacervation or phase separation technique is described.

Coacervation may be defined as a process that when solutions of two hydrophilic colloids are mixed under suitable conditions separation of liquid phase takes place. This process consists of three steps: (i) formation of three immiscible phases i.e. a liquid manufacturing vehicle phase, a core material phase and a coating material phase; (ii) deposition of the coatting material on the core; and (iii) rigidization of the coating usually by thermal, cross linking or desolvation techniques to form a microcapsule.

The substances used as coating materials include gelatin, polyvinyl alcohol, ethyl cellulose, cellulose acetate phthalate and styrene maleic anhydride. The thickness of the film can be varied according to the surface area of the material to be coated and other physical characteristics of the system. After complete process i.e. separation from the liquid manufacturing vehicle and drying, the material appears as free flowing powder which can be compressed as tablets, filled in hard gelatin capsules, suspended in a suitable liquid to form a suspension or may be converted into any other dosage forms.

Applications

Microencapsulation is used :

(1) for masking the taste of bitter drugs.
(2) for separating the incompatible ingredients.
(3) to prepare sustained action dosage froms.
(4) to protect drugs from moisture and oxidation.
(5) to prevent volatilisation of volatile substances.

14.14 Evaluation of Tablets or Standardization of Tablets

The following standards or quality control tests are carried out on compressed tablets.

1. Diameter size and shape.
2. Uniformity of weight.
3. Thickness.
4. Hardness.
5. Friability.
6. Percentage of medicament.
7. Rate of disintegration.

1. Diameter Size and Shape

The diameter size and shape of tablets depends on the die and punches selected for making the tablets. The tablets of various sizes and shapes are prepared but generally they are circular with either flat or biconvex faces.

2. Uniformity of Weight

It is desirable that all the tablets of a particular batch should be uniform in weight. If any weight variation is there, that should fall within the prescribed limits (generally ±10% for tablets weighing 120 mg. or less, ± 7.5% for tablets weighing 120 mg to 300 mg and ± 5% for tablets weighing more than 300 mg). The test is considered correct if not more than two tablets fall outside this range if 20 tablets are taken for the test and not more than one tablet falls outside this range if only ten tablets are taken for the test. The difference of weight in tablets can lead to variation in doses. Therefore all the tablets of a batch must conform to this test. For carrying out this test generally 20 tablets at random are taken and weighed. The average weight is calculated, then each tablet is weighed individually and weight noted. The weights of individual tablets are then compared with the average weight already calculated and see that not more than two tablets fall outside the range. This test is repeated after short intervals of time to ensure that tablets of required weight are produced.

3. Thickness

The thickness of a tablet can vary without any change in its weight. This is generally due to the difference of density of granules, pressure applied for compression and the speed of compression. The thickness of a tablet can be determined with the help of micrometer calipers. The thickness variation limits allowed are ±5% of the size of the tablet. The variation in thickness leads to counting and packing problems.

4. Hardness

The hardness of tablet depends on the weight of the material used, space between the upper and lower punches at the time of compression and pressure applied during compression. The hardness also depends on the nature and quantity of excipients used during formulation.

If the finished tablet is too hard, it may not disintegrate in the required period of time and if the tablet is too soft it may not withstand the handling during packing and transporting. Therefore it is very necessary to check the hardness of tablets when they are being compressed and pressure adjusted accordingly on the tablet machine.

Tablet hardness can roughly be determined by holding the tablet in between the fingers of the hand and throwing it lightly on the floor, if it does not break it indicates that proper hardness has been obtained. A number of hardness testers are used for determining the tablet hardness but Monsanto hardness testers and Pfizer hardness testers are commonly used.

(a) Monsanto Hardness Tester

It is a small, portable hardness tester which was manufactured and introduced by Monsanto Chemical Company. It consists of a spring which can be compressed by moving the screw knob forward.

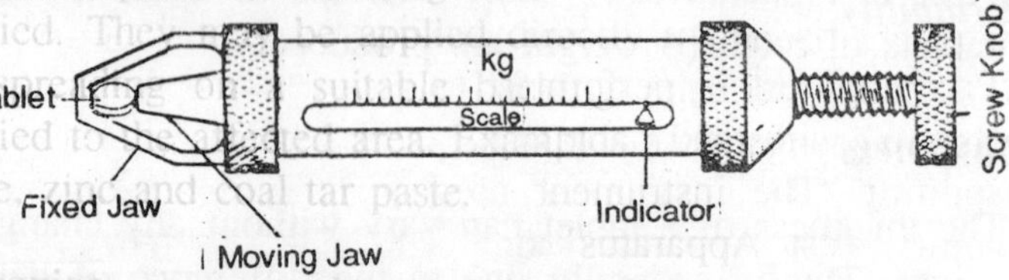

Fig. 14.9 Monsanto tablet hardness tester

The tablet to be tested is held between a fixed and a moving jaw and reading of the indicator adjusted to zero. The force applied to the edge of the tablet is gradually increased by moving the screw knob forward until the tablet breaks. The reading is noted from the scale which indicates the pressure required in kg or lb to break the tablet. Hardness of 4 kg is considered suitable for handling the tablets. Hardness of 6 kg or more will produce tablets of highly compact nature.

(b) Pfizer Tablet Hardness Tester

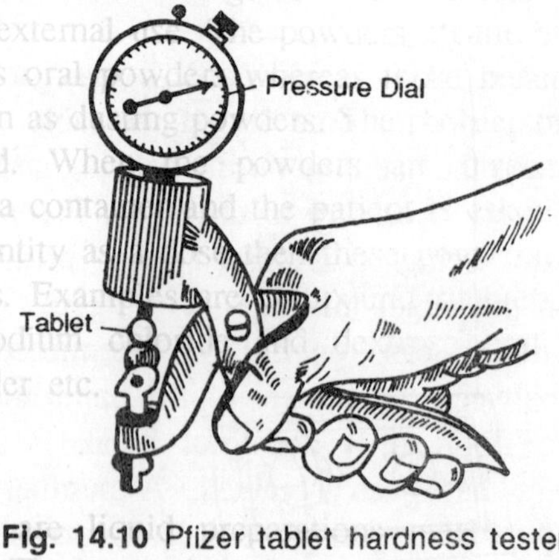

Fig. 14.10 Pfizer tablet hardness tester

It is another instrument used for testing the hardness of a tablet. It works on the principle of a plier and is similar in shape to that of a plier. It is fitted with a dial. The tablet under test is held vertically in between the jaws which are pressed with hand until the tablet breaks. The reading is noted from the needle of the pressure dial which may be expressed in kilograms or pounds of force.

5. Friability

Friability test is performed to evaluate the ability of the tablets to withstand abrasion in packing, handling and transporting. The instrument used for this test is known as 'Friability Test Apparatus' or 'Friabilator'. It consists of a plastic chamber which is divided into two parts and revolves at a speed of 25 r.p.m. A number of tablets are weighed and placed in the tumbling chamber which is rotated for four minutes or for 100 revolutions. During each revolution the tablets fall from a distance of six inches to undergo shock. After 100 revolutions the tablets are again weighed and the loss in weight indicates the friability. The acceptable limits of weight loss should not be more than 0.8 per cent.

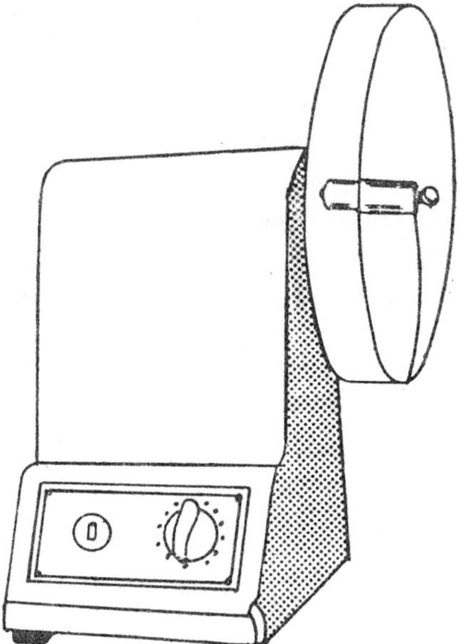

Fig. 14.11 Fibrialator

6. Percentage of Medicament

This test is performed to ensure that every tablet, coated or uncoated, must contain the stated amount of medicaments within the prescribed limits. A number of tablets from a batch are selected at random and assay procedures are carried out according to the monographs given in the official books. The results obtained must be within the prescribed percentage limits.

7. Rate of Disintegration

The disintegration test is performed to find out that within how much time the tablet disintegrates. This test is very important and necessary for all the tablets, coated or uncoated to be swallowed because the dissolution rate depends upon the time of disintegration which ultimately affects the rate of absorption of drugs.

The apparatus used for this test is known as disintegration test apparatus. This apparatus consists of a glass or plastic tube which is open at one end and the other end is fitted with a rust proof No. 10 mesh sieve.

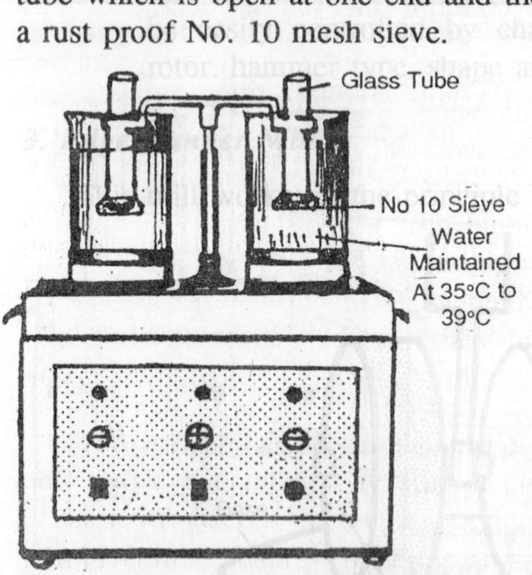

Fig. 14.12 (A) Tablet disintegration test apparatus

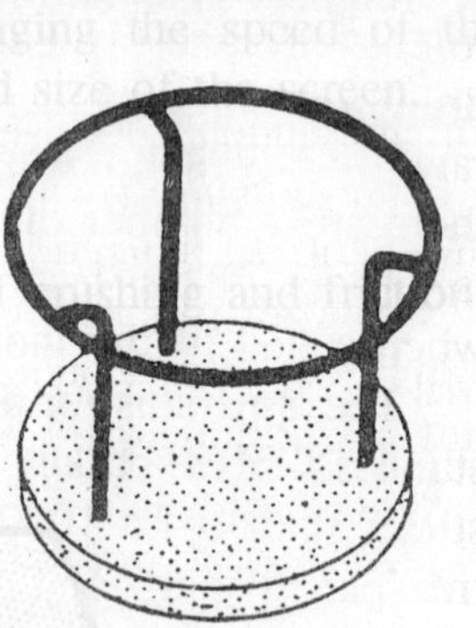

(B) Plastic disc

The tube is suspended in a bath of water or suitable liquid which is thermostatically maintained at a temperature of 37°C. The tube is allowed to move up and down at a constant rate i.e. 30 times per minute through a distance of 75 mm. The volume of the liquid and distance of movement is adjusted in such a way that at the highest point the mesh screen just breaks the surface of the liquid to give a turbulent movement to the tablets and at the lowest point the mesh screen remains about 2.5 cm. above the bottom of the container.

About five tablets are placed in the tube alongwith a plastic disk over the tablets unless otherwise stated in the monograph. The plastic disk does not allow the tablets to float and imparts a slight pressure on the tablets. The tube is allowed to move up and down and disintegration time noted when all the tablets have passed through the sieve. This time should comply with the time stated in the monograph for that tablet. The test fails if all the tablets do not pass through the sieve within specified time. Generally the disintegration time for uncoated tablets is 30 minutes and for coated tablets one hour.

8. Dissolution Test

The rate of dissolution of a solid drug plays an important role in the absorption and physiological availability of the drug in the blood stream. Therefore determination of dissolution rate of any solid drug is very necessary. For this purpose there are a number of tests available in the literature but none is official. This test is performed for tablets and capsules when stated in the individual drug monograph.

The apparatus for dissolution test consists of (i) a cylindrical stainless steel basket which is attached to the end of the stirrer shaft (ii) a 1000 ml vessel made of glass or other inert, transparent material fitted with a cover having four holes, one for the shaft of the stirrer second for placing the thermometer and remaining two for removing the samples (iii) a variable speed motor driven stirrer which can rotate at a speed of 25-150 revolutions per minute (iv) a suitable thermostatically controlled water bath to maintain the temperature of the dissolution medium at a temperature of 37°C ±0.5°C.

For performing the test a suitable volume of dissolution medium like distilled water, hydrochloric acid or phosphate buffer at a pH of 7.3 as stated in the individual monograph is filled in the glass vessel which is submerged in the water bath maintained at 37°C. The tablet or capsule to be tested is introduced in the basket and fitted in position. The motor is started and its revolutions adjusted according to monograph. The samples are withdrawn at specified intervals and filtered immediately through a suitable filter medium. Generally 5 ml sample solution is withdrawn each time which is replaced

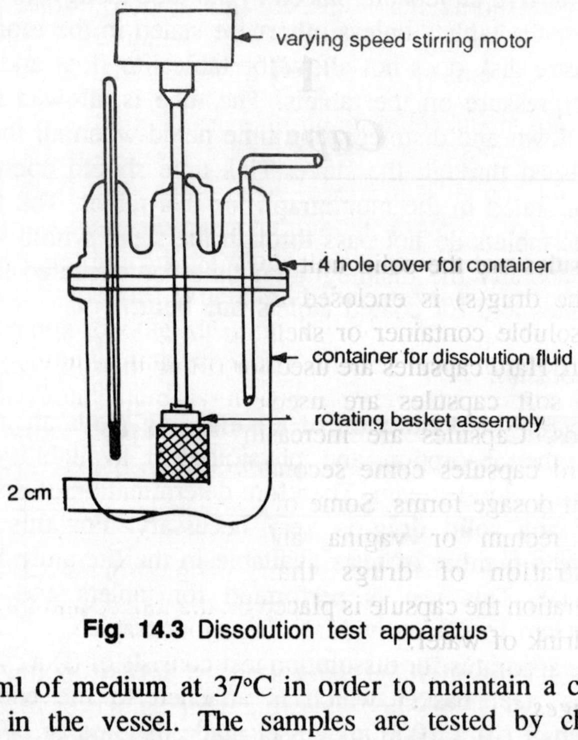

Fig. 14.3 Dissolution test apparatus

with 5 ml of medium at 37°C in order to maintain a constant volume in the vessel. The samples are tested by chemical analysis for proportion of drug dissolved which should meet the requirements as stated in the monograph.

15
Capsules

Capsules are the solid unit dosage form of medicament in which the drug(s) is enclosed in a practically tasteless, hard or soft soluble container or shell made up of a suitable form of gelatin. Hard capsules are used for filling the solid substances whereas soft capsules are used for filling the liquids and semisolids. Capsules are increasing their popularity day by day. Hard capsules come second to tablets in importance as solid unit dosage forms. Some of the capsules are administered through rectum or vagina and are convenient mode of administration of drugs than suppositories. For oral administration the capsule is placed on the tongue and swallowed with a drink of water.

Advantages

1. Capsules are tasteless, odorless and can be easily administered.
2. They are attractive in appearance.
3. The drugs having unpleasant odor and taste are enclosed in a tasteless shell.
4. They can be filled quickly and conveniently therefore the physician can change the dose and combination of drugs to suit the individual patient. This is an advantage over tablets.
5. They are economical.
6. They are easy to handle and carry.

Disadvantages

1. The drugs which are hygroscopic are not suitable for filling into capsules. They will absorb the water present in capsule shell rendering the shell very brittle and ultimately lead to crumble into pieces.
2. The concentrated solutions which require previous dilution are unsuitable for capsules because if administered as such lead to irritation in the stomach.

15.1 Hard Capsules

Hard capsules are usually made up of a base containing plasticizers and water. The base may also contain preservatives, colours, flavours and sugars. Capsule shells are made up of two cylindrical halves, one slightly large in diameter but shorter in length and the other slightly shorter in diameter and longer in length. The former is known as cap and latter as body of the capsule. The drug is filled in the narrower and longer half over which the other half is fitted as a cap.

15.2 Filling of Hard Capsules

Capsule shells are supplied in a number of sizes. The number varies from 000 to 5, the former being the largest and later the smallest. The exact amount of a medicament which can be filled in a particular size of capsule shell depends upon density of the material to be filled in. Generally the capacity varies from 600 mg to 30 mg.

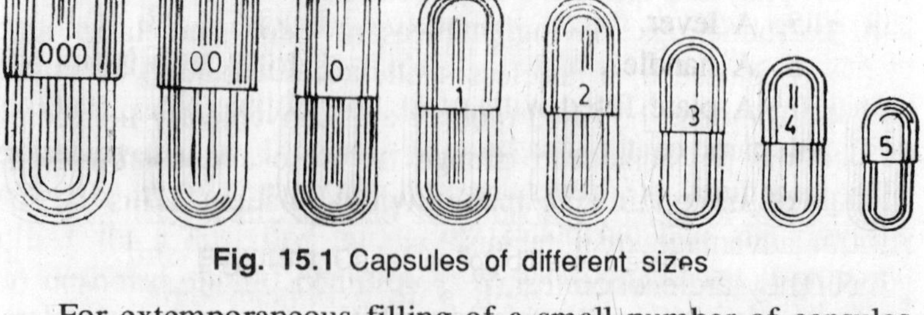

Fig. 15.1 Capsules of different sizes

For extemporaneous filling of a small number of capsules, the proper size of the capsule shell is selected which depends upon the quantity and density of the powder to be filled in. 5 to 10% excess of each ingredient is calculated just to compensate for the loss of material which remains sticking to the petle the mortar and any other surfaces which come in contact during the operation. The usual procedure is that each ingredient is weighed and finely powdered if already not in a fine powder. They are mixed together by trituration so that a uniform powder is obtained. The mixed powder is placed on a paper and spread with spatula so as to make a small pile. Remove the cap from the capsule and hold it in the left hand, press the body repeatedly into the powder until it is filled. Insert the cap on the body and weigh the capsule. While weighing each capsule of the same size must be kept in the other pan as a tare so as to get the exact quantity of drug filled in. If there are large variations in weights beyond permitted limits then it is necessary to repeat the process so as to fill the capsules with accurate quantity of drug.

15.3 Hand Operated Hard Gelatin Capsule Filling Machine

Hand operated and electrically operated machines are in practice for filling the capsules but for small and quick dispensing hand operated machines are quite economical. A hand operated hard gelatin capsule filling machine consists of the following parts.

1. A bed with 200 or 300 holes.
2. A capsule loading tray.
3. A powder tray.
4. A pin plate having 200 or 300 pins corresponding to the number of holes in the bed and capsule loading tray.
5. A lever.
6. A handle.
7. A plate fitted with rubber top.

All parts of the machine are made up of stainless steel. The machines are generally supplied with additional loading trays, beds, and pin plates with various diameters of holes so as to fill the desired size of the capsules. These machine are very simple to operate, can be easily dismantled and reassembled. Even an unskilled worker can fill the capsules without much difficulty.

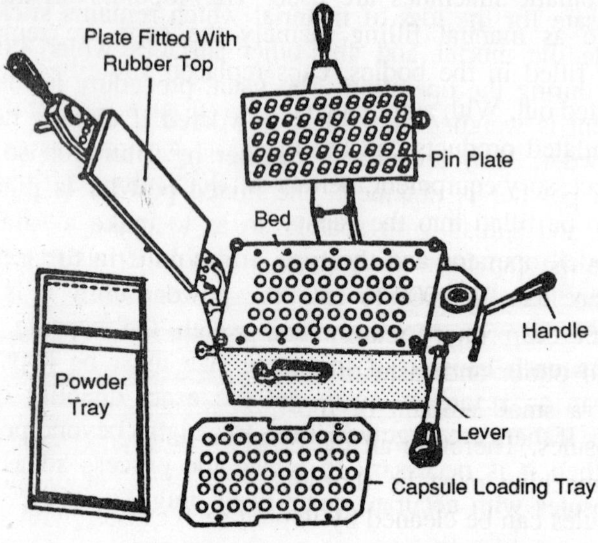

Fig. 15.2 Hand operated hard gelatin capsule filling machine

Working

The empty capsules are filled into the loading tray which is then placed over the bed. By operating the handle, the bodies of the capsules are locked and caps separated in the loading tray itself which is then removed by operating the lever. The weighed amount of the drug to be filled in the capsules is placed in powder tray already kept in position over the bed. Spread the powder with the help of a powder spreader so as to fill the bodies of the capsules uniformly. Collect excess of the powder on the platform of the powder tray. Lower the pin plate and move it downward so as to press the powder in the bodies. Remove the powder tray and place the caps holding tray in position. Press the caps with the help of plate with rubber top and operate the lever to unlock the cap and body of the capsules. Remove the loading tray and collect the filled capsules in a tray. With 200 hole machine about 5000 capsules can be filled per hour and with 300 hole machine 7500 capsules can be filled per hour.

On large scale manufacturing various types of semiautomatic and automatic machines are used. They operate on the same principle as manual filling, namely the caps are removed powder filled in the bodies, caps replaced and filled capsules are ejected out. With automatic capsule filling machines powders or granulated products can be filled into hard gelatin capsules. With accessory equipment, pellets or tablets along with powders can also be filled into the capsules. Depending upon the make and model, operator and the type of the materials to be filled, a machine can fill 9000 to 150,000 capsules per hour.

Since the primary reason of filling the drug in capsules is to avoid odour and taste of the drug. The whole aim is lost even if a small amount of the drug remains sticking outside the capsules. Therefore all the capsules whether filled by hand or by machine must be thoroughly cleaned. Small quantities of capsules can be cleaned by wiping each capsule with surgical gauze or clean cloth. On large scale they can be rolled lightly in the folds of a clean towel or cloth forward and backward until cleaned. Still another method is to rotate or shake gently the capsules with granular sodium chloride contained in a container. Then the sticking sodium chloride is removed by rolling them on a clean cloth surface.

The cleaned capsules may be polished by rolling them in a towel which has been previously sprinkled lightly with liquid paraffin. This gives very good shine to the capsules.

15.4 Difficulties in Filling the Capsules

1. Deliquescent or Hygroscopic Powders

A gelatin capsule contains water which is extracted or taken up by a hygroscopic drug and renders the capsule very brittle which leads to cracking of the capsule. The addition of an absorbent like magnesium carbonate, heavy magnesium oxide or light magnesium oxide overcomes this difficulty provided the capsules are packed in tightly closed glass capsule vials.

2. Eutectic Mixtures

Certain substances when mixed together tend to liquefy or form a pasty mass due to the formation of a mixture which has a lower melting point than room temperature. For filling these types of substances each troublesome ingredient is mixed with an absorbent separately then mixed together and filled in capsules. The absorbents used are magnesium oxide and kaolin. Heavy magnesium oxide is less effective. The use of heavy and light magnesium oxide is restricted because it forms a very hard cement like mass which passes through the G.I.T. without disintegration. But this type of mass is not formed when magnesium carbonate is used as an absorbent.

Another method in dealing with such type of difficulty is that the substances are mixed together so as to form a eutectic mixture, then an absorbent like magnesium carbonate or kaolin is added.

3. Addition of Inert Powders

When the quantity of the drug to be filled in capsules is very small and it is not possible to fill this much small amount in capsules then inert substance or a diluent is added so as to increase the bulk of the powder which can be filled easily in capsules. Generally smallest capsule requires at least 65 mg of the substance to fill it.

4. Filling of Granular Powders

Some powders which lack adhesiveness and most granular powders are difficult to fill in the capsules by punch method because they are not compressible and flow out of the capsule as soon as they are lifted from the pile of the powder into which they are punched. To overcome this difficulty the non-adhesive powders should be moistened with alcohol and the granular powders should be reduced to powder before filling into capsules.

5. Use of Two Capsules

Some of the manufacturers separate the incompatible ingredients of the formulation by placing one of the ingredients in smaller capsule and then placing this smaller capsule in a larger capsule containing the other ingredients of the formulation.

6. Liquids

Oils and liquids which will not dissolve gelatin may be filled into hard gelatin capsules. A measured quantity of the liquid is filled in the body of the capsule and the cap, the lower portion of which has been moistened with hot water is placed over the body with a rotary motion so as to seal the capsule.

When the quantity of the liquid to be incorporated is small, it is first mixed with an inert absorbent which is then added to another ingredient, mixed thoroughly and filled into capsules in the usual manner.

Viscous liquids and semisolids are mixed with an absorbent like powdered glycyrrhiza so as to form a soft mass. This soft mass is cut into desired number of pieces which are then put into capsules.

15.5 Soft Capsules

These capsules are soft and elastic in nature which are prepared from gelatin and water to which glycerin, sorbitol or propylene glycol has been added as a plasticizer which make the capsules flexible. They usually contain a preservative to pevent the growth of bacteria and fungi. These capsules are available in a number of shapes and sizes e.g. spherical , ovoid, cylindrical and tubes. The spherical capsules are also known as "pearls". The contents of the soft capsules may very from 0.1 ml to 30 ml.

The soft gelatin capsules differ from hard capsules that the latter are manufactured in two stepes where the shells are made on one type of machine and filling is done on another machine. Whereas soft capsules are formed and filled in one continuous operation on semi-automatic and automatic machines. They are hermetically sealed.

The capsules are used for filling liquids and semi-solids. Vitamin preparations such as halibut liver oil, vitamin A and

D and multivitamins are conveniently dispensed in soft capsules. They are also used for containing eye, ear, nose and throat preparations. Ophthalmic ointments are frequently packed in unit dose capsules. They are also being used as substitutes for suppositories. Now a days soft capsules are also used for packing cosmetics, flavours and food concentrates.

15.6 Preparation of Soft Capsules

Soft capsules are generally manufactured by two methods:
(1) Plate process.
(2) Rotary die process.

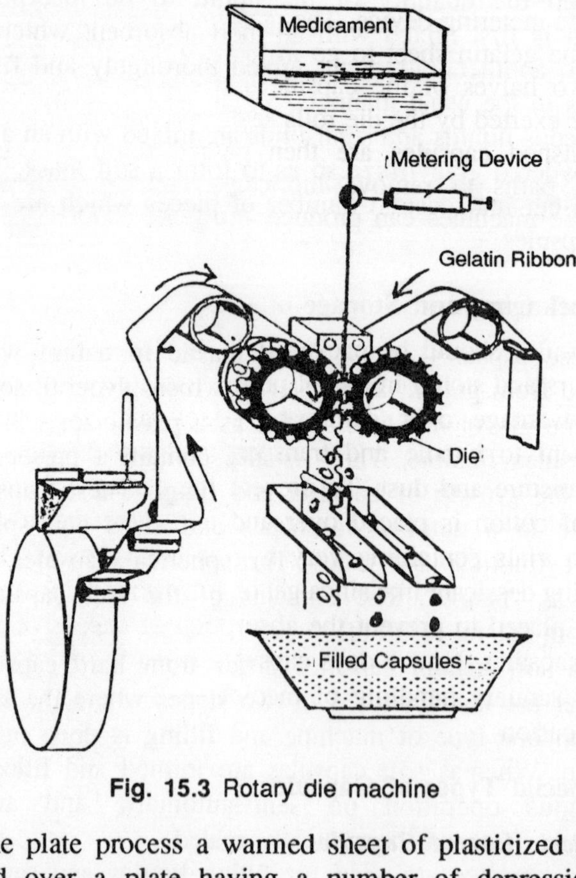

Fig. 15.3 Rotary die machine

In the plate process a warmed sheet of plasticized gelatin is placed over a plate having a number of depressions or moulds , the sheet is drawn into these depressions by applying vacuum. A measured quantity of liquid medicament is poured over it, then another sheet of gelatin is placed on it. Over this another plate of the mould is placed and the pressure is then applied to the combined plates. The capsules are then simultaneously shaped, filled, sealed and cut into individual units.

In the rotary die process filled capsules are produced continuously and automatically. Two continuous sheets of gelatin are supplied to the two die rolls of the machine which has a number of matching dies and rotate at the same speed and in the opposite direction. As the gelatin sheets comes in between the rollers the material to be filled in is injected through a metering device. The pressure exerted by the material forces the gelatin sheet to go in the cavities of the die rolls to form two halves of the capsule and fill them. The heat and pressure exerted by the die rolls seals and cuts out the capsules. The finished capsules are then passed through a series of naphtha baths to remove lubricants and then dried. These rotary die machines can produce 25000 to 30000 capsules per hour.

15.7 Packaging and Storage of Capsules

Capsules should be packed in well closed glass or plastic containers and stored in a cool place. These types of containers have advantage over cardboard boxes that they are more convenient to handle and transport and protect the capsules from moisture and dust. To prevent the capsules from rattling a tuft of cotton is placed over and under the capsules in the vials. In vials containing very hygroscopic capsules a packet containing dessicant like silica gel or anhydrous calcium chloride may be placed to prevent the absorption of excessive moisture by the capsules. Now a days capsules are strip packaged which provide sanitary handling of medicines, ease in counting and identification

15.8 Special Types of Capsules

(a) Enteric Coated Capsules

An enteric coated capsule does not disintegrate in the stomach or acidic medium but breaks up in the intestine or alkaline medium. They are given special type of treatment or coating which makes the medicine to pass unchanged through the stomach but set free in the intestine. Enteric coating may be given to following categories of drugs:

1. Which cause irritation to the gastric mucosa and lead to nausea and vomiting.
2. Which interfere with digestion e.g. tannins, silver nitrate and other salts of heavy metals .
3. Which are unstable in the gastric fluids.
4. Which are specially needed for treatment of intestine e. g. santonin, extract male fern etc.
5. Which are required to produce delayed action of the drug.

Formaldehyde, cellulose acetate phthalate and mixture of waxes with fatty acids or their esters are used for enteric coating of capsules. For extemporaneous enteric coating of capsules cellulose acetate phthalate (cellacephate) is widely used . The capsules are dropped in a 10% solution of cellulose acetate phthalate in acetone, they are removed with forceps and excess of the liquid is removed. The capsules are dried on a muslin strainer then second and third coats are applied after thorough drying each time.

(b) Sustained Release Capsules

These types of capsules release the drug slowly and continuously for a prolonged duration of action, thus maintaining a minimum effective concentration (MEC) of the drug in the blood at a constant level throughout the treatment period. Whereas in the conventional therapy i.e. administration of the drug in divided doses at specified intervals of time, a constant blood concentration is not maintained and there is considerable fluctuation in drug concentration.

The finely powdered drug is converted into pellets of suitable size (1-2 mm in diameter). These pellets are divided into a number of groups (generally 10 groups). The first group is kept untreated to produce rapid therapeutic effect and the other groups are coated with selected materials one by one to produce thickness of varying degrees. This can be done by giving two coatings to the 2nd group, 3 coatings to the 3rd group, four to the fourth group and so on. The total thickness of these coatings should be about 0.1 mm. All these groups i.e. coated and uncoated are then mixed together and filled into capsules. For coating, the materials may include cellulose esters, fats, keratin, gluten, mixtures of bees wax, carnauba wax with glyceryl monostearate.

(c) Rectal Capsules

Soft gelatin capsules may be used as substitutes for rectal and vaginal suppositories. Various shapes and sizes are used for this purpose. They are generally wider at one end which is inserted first, the movement of the sphincter muscles forces the capsules forward into the rectum. Liquids or solids can be filled into rectal capsules but the base in which the medicament have been incorporated must be non-toxic, non-irritant and compatible with the capsule shell.

(d) Capsules for Packing of Ophthalmic Ointments

It is very important that the ophthalmic ointments should be sterile and free from irritant effect. Therefore they must be packed in such a manner that the product remains sterile until whole of it is used up. The best method to keep the preparation free from contamination during use is to pack it in single dose containers. Now a days soft gelatin capsules are very commonly used for filling ophthalmic ointments. These capsules are meant for single application to the eye. Just before application, the capsule is punctured with a sterile needle, the contents instilled into the eye and the shell discarded.

15.9 Standardization of Capsules

Whether capsules are produced on a small or large scale all of them are required to pass not only the disintegration test, weight variation test and percentage of medicament test but a visual inspection must be made as they roll off the capsule machine onto a conveyor belt regarding uniformity in shape, size, colour and filling. As the capsules move in front of the inspectors the visibly defective or suspected of being less than perfect are picked out. If the number of defective capsules is large it may be due to some fault in the capsule filling machine which must be corrected.

The hard and soft gelatin capsules should be subjected to following tests for their standardization:

1. Shape and size.
2. Colour.
3. Thickness of capsule shell.
4. Leaking test for semi-solid and liquid ingredients from soft capsules.
5. Disintegration test.
6. Weight variation test.
7. Percentage of medicament test.

In official books the following quality control tests are recommended for capsules:

(a) Disintegration test

For performing disintegration test on capsules the tablet disintegration test apparatus is used but the guiding disc may not be used except that the capsules float on top of the water. One capsule is placed in each tube which are then suspended in the beakers to move up and down for 30 minutes, unless otherwise stated in the monograph. The capsules pass the test if no residue of drug or other than fragments of shell remains on No.10 mesh screen of the tubes.

(b) Weight Variation Test

20 capsules are taken at random and weighed. Their average weight is calculated. then each capsule is weighed individually and their weight noted. The capsules pass the test if the weight of individual capsule falls within 90-110% of the average weight. If this requirement is not met, then the weight of the contents for each individual capsule is determined and compared with the average weight of contents. The contents from the shells can be removed just by emptying or with the help of small brush. From soft gelatin capsules the contents are removed by squeezing the shells which has been carefully cut. The remainder contents are removed by washing with a suitable

solvent. After drying the shells, they are weighed and the content weights of the individual capsules are calculated. The requirements are met if (a) not more than 2 of the differences are greater than 10% of the average net content and (b) in no case the difference is greater than 25%.

(c) Contents Uniformity Test

This test is applicable to all capsules which are meant for oral administration. For this test a sample of the contents is assayed as described in individual monographs and the values calculated which must comply with the prescribed standards.

16
Immunity and Immunological Preparations

Immunology is the study of immunity and preparations used to produce immunity are called immunological preparations. All immunological preparations are biological products which are administered parenterally to avoid inactivation of the preparation on oral administration. The exception is poliomyelitis vaccine which is administered orally. It contains living viruses which can multiply in the gut.

16.1 Immunity

The infection or disease in human beings or animals is caused by the invasion of pathogenic microorganisms. The power of the body to resist the effects of invasion of pathogenic microorganisms is known as immunity and lack of power of the body to resist infection is called susceptibility.

There are a number of factors which are responsible for immunity but phagocytosis and antibody formation are most important.

(1) Phagocytosis Phagocytosis may be defined as the ingestion of microorganisms by certain cells of the body whereby they are rendered harmless. Phagocytosis is caused by (1) white blood corpuscles (W.B.C.) and the (2) cells of the reticuloendothelial system. The white blood cells freely float in the blood and are carried continuously to all the tissues. When the microorganisms enter the body, more and more

W.B.C. collect at the site of infection and ingest the invading bacteria, rendering them harmless. The cells of the reticuloendothelial system present in the blood spaces of liver and spleen ingest the microorganisms when the blood stream passes through liver and spleen and render the microorganisms harmless which are then carried to lungs where they are disintegrated.

(2) Antibody Production The body does not depend only on the process of phagocytosis for the destruction of pathogenic microorganisms. It produces other substances known as antibodies which destroy the pathogenic microorganisms and their toxins. Anybodies are highly specific in their nature and attack either microorganisms or toxins.

Antibodies may be defined as the substances produced in the body on the invasion of pathogenic microorganisms either to destroy these pathogenic microorganisms or their toxins.

16.2 Types of Immunity

Immunity may be classified as follows:

Immunity

- 1. Natural immunity (God gifted)
  - (a) Species
  - (b) Race
  - (c) Individual
  - (d) Age
- 2. Acquired immunity (acquired due to antibodies production)
  - (a) Active (slowly produced but long lasting)
    - (i) Naturally acquired (after infection)
    - (ii) Artificially acquired (due to administration of vaccines or antigens)
  - (b) Passive (Quickly produced but short lived)
    - (i) Naturally acquired (from mother through placenta)
    - (ii) Artificially acquired (by administration of serum preparations)

1. *Natural Immunity*

It is God gifted immunity which exerts resistance to disease. It differs between species, races, individuals and ages.

(a) Species

Certain species are immune to some diseases whereas others are not. For example man is susceptible but fowls are not; tuberculosis is very fatal to guinea-pigs but is not so fatal to man.

(b) Races

Negroes have high resistance to yellow fever whereas white men are susceptible to it.

(c) Individuals

It is well known that some persons are more resistant to cold and skin infections than others.

(d) Age

Most of the children between 2-5 years of age group are susceptible to diphtheria whereas most adults are immune to it.

2. *Acquired Immunity*

Natural immunity is not sufficient to protect the body from microbial diseases therefore additional immunity is acquired either by the stimulation of the antibody producing cells of the body (active immunity) or by introducing antibodies formed from another person or animal (passive immunity)

(a) Active Immunity

Active immunity is developed in an individual due to the formation of antibodies on the introduction of antigenic substances in the body. It may be naturally acquired or artificially stimulated.

(1) Naturally acquired active immunity It is acquired as a result of natural infection produced by pathogenic micro-organisms. There may or may not be a clinically recognisable disease. When a patient recovers from certain diseases like diphtheria, small-pox, poliomyelitis, he is left with a high degree of immunity which may last for the whole life, however after influenza, pneumonia and gonorrhea, immunity produced is short lived. Similarly children living in slum areas acquire immunity against a number of diseases because they are exposed to such diseases time and again.

(2) Artificially acquired active immunity This type of immunity is acquired by the administration of specific vaccines or toxoids. When these antigenic substances are introduced into the body, they stimulate the body to produce antibodies. Thus body develops its own defence against pathogenic microorganisms.

(b) Passive Immunity

This type of immunity is produced by the introduction of already formed antibodies into the body of an individual. These antibodies may have been developed in another individual or even in another species. Though passive immunity is rapidly produced but it is not long lasting. Passive immunity may be naturally acquired or artificially produced.

(1) Naturally acquired passive immunity In this type of immunity the antibodies are transmitted from the mother to the foetus through the placental blood. This imparts immunity to the infant for several months. Antibodies for chickenpox, diphtheria, measles and scarlet fever are transmitted in this way, that is why the infant shows high resistance against these diseases only for about six months after which this resistance is lost.

(2) Artificially produced passive immunity This type of immunity is produced by injecting antibody-containing preparations known as antisera, sera or immune sera. The antibodies are first produced in an animal usually a horse or occasionally some other person and then injected into the concerned person.

16.3 Related Terms Used in Immunity

1. *Pathogens* these are the infection causing micro-organisms.

2. *Antigens* these are the substances which stimulate the body to produce antibodies.

3. *Antibodies* these are the substances formed in the body in response to stimulation by antigens.

4. *Toxins* these are the poisonous substances produced by pathogenic microorganisms and lead to infection or disease in man or animals.

5. *Exotoxins* these are the toxins which can diffuse freely through the bacterial cell wall into the blood or the medium in which the microorganisms are growing.

6. *Endotoxins* these are the toxins which cannot diffuse through the bacterial cell wall and are retained within the bacteria. They are released only when the cells die and start disintegrating.

7. *Antitoxins* these are the substances containing antibodies produced by the blood, which specifically neutralise the toxins produced by particular microorganisms.

8. *Sera or immune sera* a clear fluid which separates from blood when it clots is known as serum. When a serum contains antitoxic antibodies it is known as antitoxic serum. They are usually obtained from animals but sometimes from human serum also.

9. *Toxoids* these are the toxins whose toxicity has been removed by gentle heat or by chemical treatment but their antigenic properties are retained e.g. tetanus toxoid and staphylococcus toxoid.

10. *Vaccines* these are the substances which are administered in the body to produce resistance against infectious diseases. They are mainly used as prophylactic treatment. Vaccines may contain living, attenuated or killed bacteria, viruses or rickettsia.

Forms of Vaccines

(1) Simple vaccines These vaccines contain only one species of microorganisms

(2) Mixed vaccines These vaccines contain two or more than two species of microorganisms.

(3) Univalent vaccines These vaccines contain only one strain of a species.

(4) Polyvalent vaccines These vaccines contain two or more strains of the same species of microorganisms.

16.4 Immunological Preparations

These are the substances or agents which are used to produce immunity in an individual. They are mainly used for the prevention of diseases e.g. vaccines. They are also used for the treatment of diseases e.g. antiserums; and also for diagnostic purposes e.g. bacterial toxins.

16.5 Classification of Immunological Preparations

The immunological preparations may be classified as follows:

1. Preparations producing active immunity
   (a) Vaccines containing living bacteria e.g. B.C.G. vaccine.
   (b) Vaccines containing dead bacteria e.g. cholera, pertussis, plague and typhoid vaccine.
   (c) Vaccines containing killed rickettesia e.g. typhus vaccine.
   (d) Vaccines containing living viruses e.g. measles, small-pox, poliomyelitis and yellow fever.
   (e) Vaccines containing toxoids e.g. diphtheria, tetanus and staphylococcus.
2. Diagnostic preparations containing bacterial toxins used for schick test and tuberculin test.
3. Preparations containing antibodies (antitoxin and antiserum) used to produce passive immunity.

1. Preparations Producing Active Immunity

Active immunity is produced by injecting antigens into the body which stimulate the production of antibodies. Antigens are administered in the form of vaccines. Active immunity is slowly developed but lasts for a long time. To produce a desired level of antibodies in the body, a number of injections of vaccines will have to be administered at specified intervals. The first injection of vaccines produces a low level of immunity. Active immunization is a prophylactic measure used to protect an individual against a particular infective disease.

Bacterial Vaccines

(a) Vaccines containing living organisms e.g. B.C.G. vaccine or Bacillus Calmette Guerin vaccine

This vaccine was developed by two French scientists, Calmette and Guerin in 1906. It is a suspension of living cells of a strain of Mycobacterium tuberculosis known as the bacillus of Calmette and Guerin.

Preparation It is prepared by growing the bacilli Mycobacterium tuberculosis on a suitable medium for not more than 14 days. The culture is then transferred to a sterile liquid which prevents the further growth but preserves the viability and antigenicity of the vaccine . The vaccine so prepared is transferred, under aseptic conditions, to sterile glass containers and sealed immediately .

B.C.G. vaccine is available both in a liquid and a freeze dried form. The latter is reconstituted immediately before use which should be used within 2 hours after its reconstitution and the unused portion must be discarded. The dried vaccine retains its potency for one year if stored at a temperature of 2°C to 10°C. The liquid vaccine gets deteriorated easily, even if stored at a low temperature therefore must be used within 14 days from the date of its manufacture. Due to this reason this vaccine cannot be tested for its toxic effects because atleast six weeks time is required for its testing therefore the vaccine is supplied without testing, hence if any untoward reactions are observed after its use further use of this batch of vaccine must be stopped immediately.

Uses

This vaccine is used as an immunizing agent against tuberculosis.

(b) Vaccines containing dead bacteria e. g. cholera, pertussis, plague and typhoid vaccine

(i) **Cholera vaccine** It is a sterile suspension of killed strains of Cholera vibrio (Vibrio cholerae) in a sodium chloride injection or other suitable diluent. It is prepared from equal portions of suspensions of Inaba and Ogawa strains of Cholera vibrio, which are grown separately. The bacteria are killed either by heating the suspension at 56°C for one hour or by treating it with a bactericide. The number of killed bacteria which should not be less then 8000 million bacteria in 1 ml. The suspension is sterilized by suitable method and then distributed in sterile ampoules or vials which are sealed immediately.

Uses

It is used for prophylactic immunization against cholera. Its effect remains for 3-6 months. It is given by subcutaneous or intramuscular injection.

(ii) **Pertussis vaccine** It is a sterile suspension of killed strains of Pertussis bacilli (Bordetella pertussis) in a sodium chloride injection or other suitable diluent. It is prepared by growing one or more strains of B.pertussis on a suitable liquid medium for 24 to 72 hours. The bacteria are killed by heating the suspension at 56°C or by adding a suitable bactericide. The suspension is centrifuged, the supernatant liquid is discarded and the deposited bacteria are suspended in a sodium chloride injection or other suitable diluent isotonic with blood. The suspension at this stage is very concentrated which is kept in the cold for about three months to eliminate abnormal toxicity. This concentrated suspension is then diluted with sodium chloride injection or other suitable diluent to get final dilution of the preparation. The number of killed bacteria are counted in the suspension which should not be less than 20000 million bacteria in 1 ml.

Uses

It is used for active immunization of children against whooping cough. It is given by subcutaneous injection.

(iii) **Plague vaccine** It is a sterile suspension of killed strains of Plague bacilli(Pasteurella pestis) in isotonic sodium chloride solution or other suitable diluent. It is prepared similar to pertussis vaccine by growing a strain of P. pestis on a suitable media. Plague vaccine contains 3000 million bacteria in 1 ml.

Uses

This vaccine is used for immunization against plague. It is given by intramuscular or subcutaneous injection.

(iv) **Typhoid-** (paratyphoid A and B vaccine). It is a sterile suspension of killed strains of Salmonella typhi, S. paratyphi A, and S. paratyphi B. It is prepared similar to pertussis vaccine, from strains of S. typhi, S. paratyphi A, and S. paratyphi B grown on suitable culture media. This vaccine is also known as TAB vaccine. TABC contains S. paratyphi C in addition to TAB.

Uses

TAB vaccine is used for immunization against typhoid fever. It is given by subcutaneous injection.

(c) Vaccines containing killed rickettsia e.g. typhus vaccine

It is a suitable suspension of the killed typhus rickettsia. It may be prepared by injecting small doses of living organisms into the yolk sacs of fertile eggs which have been incubated for seven days. They are again incubated for 4 to 7 days or until the yolk sac is heavily infected. The yolk sacs are ground to liberate maximum number of rickettsia and the material is suspended in a saline or other suitable diluent isotonic with blood. The product so obtained is purified by extraction with solvent ether, to remove fatty matter from the yolk. The resultant suspension is distributed under aseptic conditions in sterile containers and sealed immediately.

Uses

This vaccine is used for immunization against diseases

and infections caused by rickettsia. It is given by subcutaneous injection.

(d) Vaccines containing living viruses e.g. smallpox, measles, poliomyelitis vaccine etc.

(i) **Smallpox vaccine** It is a liquid or dried preparation of Vaccinia virus grown on the skin of living healthy sheep or calves; or in the membranes of the chick embryo.

Method of Preparation by using Animals

A brief account of different stages involved for the preparation of smallpox vaccine is given below:

1. Selection of animals
2. Preparation for scarification
3. Scarification and inoculation
4. Incubation
5. Withdrawal of contents of pustules
6. Purification
7. Packing and storage

1. Selection of Animals

Generally living mammals e.g. calves or sheep are selected for the production of smallpox vaccine. Before selection of the animals they are kept in quarantine for 10-14 days under observation. Those proved quite healthy and free from any disease are selected for the purpose.

2. Preparation for Scarification

The selected animal is thoroughly scrubbed, washed and disinfected. Then the animals is taken to a special room where the flanks and abdomen are shaved, rescrubbed and thoroughly redisinfected.

3. Scarification and Inoculation

The prepared animal is shifted to an aseptic room where longitudinal light scratches are made on the scarified area of the abdomen and flanks, with the help of a comb like device, the scarifier; without drawing blood. This process of making light scratches on the skin of the animal is known as scarification. The scarified area is then rubbed with a seed virus of known potency, obtained from the animal previously suffering from cowpox.

4. Incubation

The inoculated area is allowed to incubate. During the next 4 to 5 days, pustules or vesicles containing the virus develop along the lines of scarification. During all this period every precaution must be taken to keep the animal and inoculated area as clean and aseptic as possible.

5. Withdrawal of Contents of Pustules

The animal is brought to the operation table and killed. A postmortem is done to confirm the absence of infectious diseases which are not detected otherwise. The abdomen and flanks are washed with sterile water and contents of pustules are withdrawn with the help of a special sharp edged instrument, with aseptic precautions.

6. Purification

The contents withdrawn are treated with glycerin, with or without some other bactericide, to kill the pathogenic microorganisms and to reduce the number of other bacterias to a very low level. The glycerin treated contents are stored for a long time at –10°C. Now a days the purification is done by extracting the contents with trichlorotrifluoroethane or other suitable protein solvent by means of centrifugation. The supernatant liquid is treated with phenol 0.4% W/V. Sufficient glycerin and peptone are added and a suitable colouring agent may also be incorporated. After purification it is stored at a temperature –10°C.

7. Filling

The purified contents are distributed in sterilized single dose capillary tubes holding 0.06 ml which are then sealed.

The sealed containers must be stored at a temperature below 0°C because it loses its potency at room temperature.

Alternative Method of Preparation using Eggs

Hen's eggs which have been incubated for twelve days are selected. A small cut of the shape of a triangle is made in the shell which is lifted up gently to expose the chorioallantoic membrane. This membrane is inoculated with seed viruses, the opened cut is sealed by replacing the flap in position and the eggs are incubated for 72 hours. After this time the shells are separated and contents added to sterile saline solution at 0°C . The material is ground to obtain a homogeneous product which is then transferred to sterile capillary tubes.

Uses

This vaccine is used for active immunization against small-pox. This is applied on the suitably scarified area of the forearm or shoulder of the individual to be vaccinated.

(ii) **Measles vaccine** Measles vaccine is of two types:

(a) Measles vaccine containing attenuated living viruses.

(b) Measles vaccine containing killed viruses (inactivated vaccine).

Generally attenuated measles vaccines has high antigenic properties than the inactive measles vaccines. The former causes severe reactions whereas the latter is almost reaction free and is a poor immunizing agent therefore it is not used alone. It is administered to reduce the reactions from the attenuated living vaccines almost four to six weeks before injecting the attenuated living vaccine.

Measles vaccines containing attenuated living viruses is an aqueous suspension of a suitable attenuated living strain of measles virus grown in chick embryo tissues only.

Measles vaccine containing killed viruses is aqueous suspension of a suitable measles virus grown in chick embryo or in monkey kidney cells. The virus are inactivated by a siutable method and may be adsorbed on aluminium hydroxide or aluminium phosphate. The resulting product will be more efficient antigen.

The measles vaccines are prepared similar to that of poliomyelitis vaccine.

Uses

This vaccine is used by injection for prophylaxis of measles.

(iii) Poliomyelitis vaccines There are two types of poliomyelitis vaccines:

(a) Poliomyelitis vaccine containing killed viruses (inactivated vaccine)

(b) Poliomyelitis vaccine containing attenuated living virus (oral vaccine)

Poliomyelitis vaccine containing killed viruses is an aqueous suspension of suitable strains of poliomyelitis virus, types 1,2 and 3 grown in cultures of monkey kidney tissues and inactivated by suitable method . It is administered by parenteral route.

Poliomyelitis vaccine containing attenuated living virus is an aqueous suspension of suitable, living attenuated strains of poliomyelitis virus type 1,2 and 3 grown in cultures of monkey kidney tissues. It is given by oral route and is the more preferred vaccine than the inactivated vaccine.

Oral poliomyelitis vaccine is prepared by using strains of poliomyelitis virus type 1,2 and 3 which are grown separately in cultures of monkey kidney tissues. For this purpose Rhesus monkeys free from tuberculosis and other communicable diseases are selected. The virus suspensions are harvested within six days of inoculation and mixed in suitable proportions and filtered through bacteria-proof filter. The filtered vaccine is tested for identity and virus concenration. The tested vaccine is filled in sterile containers.

Uses

This vaccine is used for the prophylaxis of poliomyelitis and is given by mouth.

(iv) Yellow fever vaccine Yellow fever vaccine contains an attenuated strain of yellow fever virus known as 17 D strain. It is an aqueous suspension of chick embryo tissue infected with 17 D strain virus.

For the preparation of dried vaccine of yellow fever the secondary seed virus is injected into the embryo of fertile eggs. After incubation for further 3-4 days, the embryoes are removed and mixed which are then ground and extracted with sterile water. The suspension so obtained is then centrifuged to remove cell material. The supernatant liquid is mixed with suitable stabilizer and distributed in sterile containers and freeze dried. Since this vaccine gets decomposed very quickly in the presence of oxygen therefore after freeze drying, the ampoules are immediately filled with sterile nitrogen to replace oxygen from the containers and sealed.

Use

This vaccine is used for active immunization against yellow fever.

When the vaccine is to be administered it is reconstituted from the dried vaccine with normal saline solution or any other suitable solvent so that the vaccine should be isotonic with blood. The reconstituted vaccine undergoes rapid deterioration therefore it must be used within half an hour.

(e) Vaccines containing Toxoids e.g. diphtheria, tetanus and staphylococcus

Pathogenic microorganisms produce poison or toxic substances as a byproduct of their metabolism called toxins. These toxins can't be used as antigenic substances. Their toxicity is removed either by gentle heating or by treating with certain chemicals but their antigenic properties are retained. Toxins which are detoxified are known as toxoids . They are used for the development of active immunity, examples are diphtheria vaccine , tetanus toxoid and staphylococcus toxoid.

(i) **Diphtheria vaccine** *A* toxin is first prepared by growing a suitable strain of corynebacterium diphtheriae on a liquid medium which must not be made with horse flesh or serum to prevent sensitizing reactions. After incubation at optimum temperatures until sufficient concentration of toxin is obtained, the microorganisms are collected on paper pulp and passed through bacteria proof filters. The filtrate constitutes the desired toxin.

To the toxin so obtained, formaldehyde solution (formalin) is added and the mixture is incubated at 37°C for 2-3 weeks so as to remove toxicity. This detoxicated toxin is known as Formol Toxoid (F.T.) which is unpurified form of vaccine. Now a days a number of purified products are available which are discussed as under:

(a) Alum Precipitated Toxoid (A.P.T.)

The Formol toxoid is treated with charcoal to remove colouring matter and some of the non-specific impurities. After washing and filtration to remove the charcoal, a suitable concentration of alum is added which precipitates the toxoid. The precipitates so obtained are repeatedly washed with and suspended in normal saline solution.

(b) Purified Toxoid Aluminium Phosphate(P.T.A.P.)

It is prepared by adding purified formol toxoid to a suspension of hydrated aluminum phosphate in a saline or other suitable solution isotonic with blood.

(c) Toxoid Antitoxin Floccules (T.A.F.)

It is prepared by mixing formalin treated diphtheria toxin and excess of diphtheria antitoxin. The floccules so obtained are separated, washed and suspended in saline or other suitable solution isotonic with blood. This product is known as toxoid-antitoxin floccules. It has weaker antigenic properties than alum precipitated toxoid but it rarely causes sensitization reactions, therefore, is very suitable for adults who are susceptible to A.P.T.

Uses

This vaccine is used for active immunization against diphtheria.

(ii) **Tetanus toxoid.** This is also known as tetanus vaccine and is prepared from tetanus toxin produced by the growth of Clostridium tetani on a suitable culture medium. It is of two types (i) tetanus Formol toxoid and (ii) tetanus alum precipitated toxoid. The method of preparation of these toxoids is similar to that of diphtheria Formol toxoid and diphtheria alum precipitated toxoid.

Uses

It is used for active immunization against tetanus.

(iii) **Staphylococcus toxoid.** It is a sterile filtrate prepared from a suitable strain of Staphylococcus and the alpha toxin produced is modified by treating it with formaldehyde solution and heat until the toxicity has been completely removed or reduced to a low level.

Uses

It is used for the prophylaxis of staphylococcal infections.

2. Diagnostic Preparations Containing Bacterial Toxins

These diagnostic preparations are used:

(a) to identify whether an individual is susceptible or immune to a particular infection.
(b) to determine whether a useful degree of protection has been provided or not after immunization.
(c) to indicate whether a particular disease is present in an individual or not.

The following preparations are used for diagnostic purposes:

(i) Schick test toxin.
(ii) Schick control.
(iii) Old tuberculin.

Schick test toxin and Schick control are used to identify whether an individual is susceptible or immune to diphtheria.

(i) Schick test toxin is a sterile filtrate prepared from exotoxins obtained from a suitable culture of Corynebacterium diphtheriae. It is diluted with normal saline and borax-boric acid buffer so as to stabilize its pH. The exotoxin is diluted in such a way that the test dose is contained in 0.2 ml.

(ii) Schick control is the Schick test toxin from the same batch as that used for the test which has been heated between 70°C to 85°C for not less than 5 minutes to destroy the toxin. It is used to identify whether the inflammation caused is due to test or due to substances other than toxins and to confirm whether the individual is susceptible or immune to diphtheria.

Application of the Test

These two preparations i.e. Schick test toxin and Schick control are administered on the same occasion. The test dose of toxin is injected intracutaneously into the left forearm and an equal volume of Schick control is injected into the right forearm of the individual. The site of each injection is examined after one to two days. If the left forearm into which toxin has been injected shows redness or inflammation it shows that the toxin is not neutralized and the individual is susceptible to diphtheria but if there is no redness or inflammation it shows that the person is immune. If the redness or inflammation appears it may be due to substances other than toxins which is confirmed from right forearm. If on the right forearm also there is no reaction, it shows that the person is immune but if reaction is observed the person is susceptible to diphtheria.

(iii) **Old tuberculin.** This is used to identify whether a person is suffering from tuberculosis or not. Persons suffering from tuberculosis or who have recovered from tuberculosis are extremely sensitive to tuberculin and show positive reactions.

Tuberculin was first developed by Koch and still official and prepared according to his preparation hence named old tuberculin. It is prepared by growing Mycobacterium tuberculosis on a fluid medium containing 5% glycerin at 37°C for six weeks or more to obtain abundant growth of microorganisms. Then the culture is steamed for about an hour to kill the organisms and concentrated on water bath to about 1/10th of its original volume, a preservative is added and the solution is sterilized by filtration. The final sterile product is distributed in sterile glass containers which are sealed immediately.

(iv) **Tuberculin Purified Protein Derivative (Tuberculin P.P.D.).** It is the active protein which is isolated from old tuberculin by fractional precipitation with ammonium sulphate, trichloroacetic acid or other suitable protein precipitant. This preparation has several advantages over old tuberculin that it is free from constituents of culture media, stable in dry conditions, easy to prepare in solution form and has constant composition and potency.

Tuberculin P.P.D. is available as concentrated solution, in the form of sterile tablets suitably diluted with lactose and as a freeze dried powder. It is distributed in sterile containers and sealed immediately.

3. Preparations Containing Antibodies (Antitoxin and Antiserum) Used to Produce Passive Immunity

Antibodies are the substances which are produced in response to stimulation by antigens. When a person or animal has been actively immunized either by natural or artificial means the blood contains a large number of antibodies. When the blood is withdrawn and allowed to clot, the blood cells and a clear liquid known as serum is separated which contains the antibodies. These serum containing antibodies are known as antitoxins. A serum may contain antitoxin, antibacterial or antiviral antibodies and are known as antitoxin, antibacterial or antiviral serum respectively. Antitoxin serums are commonly known as antitoxins. Generally antisera are obtained from animals (usually horses) but sometimes from human serum also. The antisera obtained from animals include diphtheria antitoxin, gas-gangrene antitoxin, antirabies serum etc. whereas those obtained from human serum include measles immune serum, mumps immune serum etc. Sometimes serum obtained from animals produce allergic reactions in human beings therefore they must be thoroughly tested before administration.

Antitoxins and antiserum are used to produce passive immunity against infective diseases. Their onset of action is rapid because 'ready made' antibodies are administered but the immunity produced lasts only for a short time. They are generally administered to those persons who have come in contact with infective disease, so as to give them immediate protection against the disease and afterwards active immunity is produced either naturally or artificially.

Diphtheria Antitoxin

It is a sterile, nonpyrogenic solution containing the specific antitoxic antibodies obtained from the serum of healthy horses and have the power of neutralizing the toxin formed by Corynebacterium diphtheriae.

Diphtheria antitoxin is produced from horses. Horses are preferred because they are large and considerable quantity of blood can be withdrawn at a time without any ill effects. Sometimes other animals e.g. goats are used to produce antitoxin for those individuals who are sensitive to horse serum.

The healthy horses are isolated for seven days and those free from infectious diseases such as glanders are selected and immunised against tetanus.

For active immunization, a pure culture of the causative organism Corynebacterium diphtheriae is obtained and a toxoid is prepared. After isolation and thorough examination of horses, the toxoid is injected into the muscles of the neck by I/m injection. The first dose of toxoid is usually not more than 5 ml which is gradually increased daily or after 1-2 days for about two months and as much as 600 ml is injected for the final dose.

After about 10 days of injection of final dose, about eight litres of blood are withdrawn aseptically into bottles containing anticoagulant solution. Similarly two more collections each about eight litres of blood are made within next eight days after which horse is given about 15 days rest. Then another course of toxoid is repeated in similar doses to stimulate further antibody production and blood collected in three batches each measuring about eight litres. Further courses of administration of toxoid and bleeding are continued for 4-5 times or till the animal stops producing satisfactory antitoxin.

After collection of the blood it is kept in the refrigerator for about two days during which cells settle down and the clear liquid is separated to which calcium chloride is added to induce clotting. The clotted material is separated from serum by filtration. A suitable bactericide (about 0.5% phenol) may be added to the filtrate, filled in suitable containers and sealed.

A dry product may be obtained by drying the filtrate at low temperature to form a powder. No bactericide may be added to the dried product.

Uses

It is used for prophylaxis and treatment of diphtheria.

Other Antitoxins

(i) Botulinum antitoxin (Clostridium botulinum)
(ii) Gas-gangrene antitoxin (Clostridium welchii) (Clostridium septicum)
(iii) Staphylococcus antitoxin (Staphylococcus aureus)
(iv) Tetanus antitoxin (Clostridium tetani) The above mentioned antitoxins are prepared by similar procedures like that of diphtheria antitoxin except that the appropriate bacterial toxin or toxoid is injected in the animal.

Antibacterial sera

Antibacterial sera are used to provide passive immunity for diseases caused by endotoxin producing bacteria. they were used against a number of diseases e.g. typhoid, pneumonia and meningitis but now these sera have been replaced by chemotherapeutic agents. No antibacterial sera is official now a days but Leptospira antiserum is included in B.P.C. This preparation is occasionally used with chemotherapeutic agents in the early treatment of spirochaetal jaundice which is also known as Weil's disease. This antiserum is not used for prophylaxis.

Antiviral sera

Antiviral sera are used to produce passive immunity and the main source of antiviral antibodies is human serum e.g. measles, German measles, etc. but rabies antiserum is prepared in horses.

Rabies antiserum

It is prepared from horses by giving a course of dead rabies virus to horses followed by a course of living virus. Then the blood is collected and the gamma-globulin fraction containing the antiviral antibodies separated.

This antiserum is highly effective in preventing rabies if administered within 24 hours of bitten by the animal. It is given along with rabies vaccine for preventing rabies if the person is bitten in a sensitive area like head and neck and specially if the animal is suspected to be rabid.

Measles Serum

For the preparation of measles serum human serum is used and not the animal serum. Three types of human immune serum have been introduced for the prevention and treatment of measles which are as follows:

(i) Convalescent measles serum
(ii) Adult measles serum
(iii) Placental extracts.

(i) **Convalescent measles serum.** Convalescent measles serum is prepared from the blood of children who are recently recovered from measles because at this time the blood contains a large number of antibodies. Serum is collected from children because they are more susceptible to measles than adults.

(ii) **Adult measles serum.** It is prepared from the blood of healthy adults who had suffered from measles in the past or in their childhood. This serum is less effective than convalescent serum.

(iii) **Placental extracts.** New born babies are immune to a number of infectious diseases like diphtheria, scarlet fever and measles due to the presence of large number of antibodies received from the mother through the placental blood. These antibodies can be separated from placental blood by different methods; which are used as measles serum and they are as potent as that of convalescent serum.

16.6 Storage of Immunological Products

Immunological products lose their potency on storage due to denaturation of antigens or antibodies by chemical reactions which are largely influenced by storage temperature. Higher the temperature larger will be deterioration and vice versa, therefore these products must be stored at a low temperature and they should be protected from sunlight as sunlight also leads to decomposition of immunological products.

Most of the bacterial vaccines, antitoxins and antisera should be stored in a refrigerator at temperatures between 2°C to 10°C, freezing should be avoided. A number of viral vaccines e.g. smallpox vaccine and poliomyelitis vaccine should be stored at or below their freezing points because they remain stable at this temperature. Antisera should be protected from light. Freeze-dried vaccines e.g. smallpox vaccines and yellow fever vaccines must be stored at a temperature of 10°C and 0°C respectively.

The recommended storage conditions and expiry dates of the immunological products are always printed on the label of the containers and these instructions must be carefully followed.

Index